A DAUGHTER'S
LAMENT
2

A DAUGHTER'S LAMENT

2

The Continuing Trials and Tribulations of a Family Caregiver

Eden Rosen

To order additional copies of this book, contact:
Xlibris Corporation
1-888-795-4274
www.Xlibris.com
Orders@Xlibris.com
14485

ACKNOWLEDGEMENTS

As with the original, I dedicate this book to the millions of family caregivers who have gone through hell fighting for their rights and their loved ones out of love.

I also dedicate "A Daughter's Lament 2" to my father because it really is a very sad period in my life.

A portion of the proceeds will be donated to various nonprofit organizations dealing with dementia or those agencies that aid family caregivers.

CONTENTS

PREFACE AND INTRODUCTION 9

CHAPTER ONE: THE CONTINUING TRIALS
     AND TRIBULATIONS 11

CHAPTER TWO: DEALING WITH DIFFICULT
     BEHAVIORS 47

CHAPTER THREE: HMO ISSUES 59

CHAPTER FOUR: IN-HOME AGENCIES:
     THE PROBLEMS CONTINUE 82

CHAPTER FIVE: LANDLORDS, TENANTS,
     AND THE NEIGHBORS 107

CHAPTER SIX: THE MOVE 123

CHAPTER SEVEN: DEALING WITH COURT 127

CHAPTER EIGHT: DEALING WITH
     THE GOVERNMENT 131

CHAPTER NINE: COMMENTS BETTER
     LEFT UNSAID 140

CHAPTER TEN: EMPLOYERS: DO THEY
     REALLY KNOW HOW TO MANAGE? 143

CHAPTER ELEVEN: THE CLOSING CHAPTER 146

PREFACE AND INTRODUCTION

I cannot sleep. It is a good time to begin the completion of the unfinished issues I left in my original book.

People with dementia become worse. They do not get better. The disease progresses. It takes its toll on both caregiver and care recipient.

The sequel starts where I stopped in December 2000. It covers many of the same issues with which I dealt in the original book but it gives different examples.

This book is important. I want to continuously raise awareness of what it means to be a caregiver to a cognitively impaired adult.

I hope by the time the general public, professional caregivers, etc. read this, they will have a greater understanding of the tasks we perform on a 24/7/365 basis.

CHAPTER ONE

THE CONTINUING TRIALS
AND TRIBULATIONS

My father missed the chair and landed on the floor. This is not the first time. Fortunately, he did not get hurt. The chair made a very loud noise when it banged against the wall.

Since my original book, several times, I have seen and heard my father ask for his Mama. Tonight, he kept telling me he wanted to go outside. I asked him where he wanted to go. He said he wanted to see Mama. He wanted to go home. I said, "You miss Mama very much, don't you?" He said yes and I almost cried.

I do not know about you but this breaks my heart. I cannot change what is happening to my father. I can only change my reaction to the disease and its effects. However, changing my reaction does not make things any easier. I find it difficult watching my father asking for his Mama. I think it always will bother me.

I also find it difficult to see my father hit himself on the head. I asked him why he was hitting himself on the head. He said that there are a lot of flies around his head. In reality, there were no flies.

Although there are drugs to control hallucinations, I would rather not have the doctors give him anything for the hallucinations. My father experienced too many problems while on psychotropic medication.

Seeing my father hallucinate is horrible but dealing with the adverse effects of the psychotropic drugs is worse in my father's case. (Refer to original book).

One day, my father ordered me to sit down. He gave me the order approximately six times. He told me if I did not sit, I would be beaten by the prisoners. He believed we were being held captive. Finally, he moved onto something else.

He told me to look under the blanket because he thought a child was underneath. He also believed the child was being smothered by the blanket.

Then, he asked me to check one of the paintings hanging on my wall. I have to see if it is the same painting. In order to get him to move onto something else, I had to check the painting.

Dad is very restless this morning. At 3:30a.m., he woke me. I do not know what he is feeling. I cannot ferret it out of him. He told me to leave him alone. I told him I was going back to bed. I did. At 5:30a.m., I awoke and found him in the exact position in which I left him. I asked him what was wrong. This time, he told me he had to get a shipment out to this guy. He thought the bathroom was the factory. Somehow, I managed to convince him that the shipment could go out later and to go back to bed. Fifteen minutes later, he was back under the covers and asleep.

Dad wanted to go home. He wanted me to go home with him. He became obsessed with wanting to go home. He even believed his wife was waiting for him at home. For twenty minutes, he kept yelling help and telling me he wanted to go home. Finally, after twenty minutes which seemed like an eternity, he gave up and dozed off for a nap. This is the only time I have to accomplish my tasks.

He woke up and after some very tense moments, when he would not allow me to change him, he finally went to bed for the night. (See chapter on difficult behaviors).

However, he awoke at 4:30a.m, 5:30a.m., and 6:00a.m. He needed to send a shipment to New England. I convinced him it was too early and he returned to bed.

Sometimes, my father shows he still has a sense of humor. A few days ago I told him I was going bye-bye. He said, "Where are you bye-byeing?" I told him I had to run errands.

People who meet him, when he is in a good mood, think he is just so cute and charming. He is cute until he repeats the same questions, becomes agitated, threatens to harm me, or becomes constipated. Then, he is not so cute.

The disease has its ups and downs. Things do not get better, just worse.

As the disease progresses, my father may or may not continue to recognize me. I know there have been several times when he does not know who I am. Also, as the disease progresses, someone with dementia may not recognize himself or herself in the mirror.

Recently, I showed my father a picture of him from 24 years ago with our former two dogs. He recognized himself. However, when he looked in the mirror this particular night, he asked me about the man in the mirror. However, the next morning, as he peered into the mirror, he knew who was the man in the mirror.

My father is not feeling too well. As expected, he is grumpy and restless. I had to walk him to the bathroom many times. He would sit on the couch and yell help. I could not get any work accomplished. My patience began to wane. I found it very diffi-cult to keep running back and forth to the sad tune of, "Help, help, help" every few seconds. I had to hide for a few minutes to pull myself together. Once I did, I began to feel a little better and more able to cope.

To those of you who have judged me without ever walking a mile in my shoes, try being a caregiver to a loved one with Alzheimer's or vascular dementia. Then tell me what emotions and behaviors you have experienced. I think you will not be so quick to judge someone else who is a family caregiver.

My father felt more comfortable last night. Even with the fiber and stool softeners, he still experienced elimination prob-lems. For most of the night, I took him back and forth to the bathroom numerous times. Finally, at approximately 3:00a.m. he went back to the bathroom. I knew he would eliminate some more. However, I did not know when he would have to make another trip to the bathroom. He went back to the couch and fell soundly asleep.

I could not sleep. I went to bed approximately 5:40a.m. and awoke 8:15a.m., certainly not ready for another day.

The caregiver came at 9:30a.m. and off I ran to do what I needed to accomplish.

As I keep saying, most people do not have a clue. How can anybody say that caring for a person with vascular dementia is the same as raising a child? It is because they do not understand.

It is January, 2001. My father awoke from a nap yelling "Help." I walked over to him and asked him what was wrong. He became very sad and said, "22 parties and I cannot go to one of them." I thought he was going to cry. I told him that our former neighbor was moving and after she moved she was going to come here with wine, cheese, and fruit. We were going to have a three person party. Then, I hugged him and he settled down.

I have a difficult time watching my father lose his memory and his functions. I find it heartbreaking.

I tried fixing and working on my computer. I had problems. My father kept calling "Help" every minute. Most of the time he did not need any help. I think he felt lonely. However, I had to stop what I was doing and see to him. I felt frustrated and lost my patience because I was on a long distance call to the computer technician. At one point, he did need help going to the bathroom.

I also became frustrated with my computer, the manufacturer and the employees. One employee understood. I had to put her on speaker and she heard my father in the background. She said, "God bless you." I told her that I needed all the help I could obtain.

I took a break from the computer because it gave me a headache. Later, in the evening, I returned to do more work on the computer. As soon as I started, he began to yell "Help." He did not stop. Finally, he admitted he felt lonely.

Unfortunately, I could not drop everything and keep him company on the couch. The computer is approximately 10 feet from him but he needed to be closer. He continued calling "Help." I had to tell him several times I would be there in a few minutes. The only problem with that is my father has lost the ability to determine what I mean when I say a few minutes. I could not think of anything else to say or do. Anyway, I told him six times that I would be there soon.

I finished my work, shut down the computer, and went to keep him company. He became happy and complacent.

The next time he kept yelling "Help" and admitted he felt lonely, I put out a chair within arms length of the computer. I had him sit on the chair. He sat for a few minutes, got up, and went to the couch. He did this several times.

Later, that night, he kept asking for his shoes. He believed somebody stole them. I had to show him where they were located. He became more complacent and settled.

However, a few minutes later, I was cleaning the kitchen. He kept telling me to shut off the light in the kitchen. I had to tell him several times I would shut off the light when I was finished. He finally said all right.

Then, my father asked me three times what I was doing. I said, "Cleaning." A few seconds later, he asked me, "What's that?" I did not have a clue about what he was talking. I guessed. He was either talking about the laundry basket or the vacuum cleaner. He finally pointed to the basket. I said laundry. For whatever reason telling him it was a laundry basket seemed to pacify him.

Later that evening, my father started to sing. He was not loud but I wanted to get him to stop singing. He stopped about ten minutes later.

Approximately fifteen minutes later, he wanted me to shut off the night light in the bathroom. He thought it was a fire burning. He whined and moaned about it being lit. I explained as many times as I needed that it was a night light and it would help him find his way to the bathroom. It took awhile to sink in, but he finally understood. He became calmer.

He was restless all night, finally falling asleep at 5:30a.m. Later that morning, I made breakfast. Thirty minutes afterward, he forgot he ate.

Dad awoke at 4:15a.m. He was very hyper. He kept asking for his shoes. He wanted to put them on and go outside. He told me his father was waiting for him down the street.

My father would not go back to bed. He kept pacing back and forth. After I walked him around the apartment, I asked if he felt hungry. He said yes. I made him some cereal. After eating, he got into his bed and went to sleep. It was 4:45a.m.

He woke up several times between 4:45a.m. and 8:45a.m., waking me up in the process.

The above incidents are part and parcel of a very horrible disease.

I finally got out of bed for good about 9:30a.m. but not before the toddler in this building ran around the upstairs walkway three times. If that was not enough, my upstairs neighbors played their TV until 1:00a.m.

My job is difficult enough without inconsiderate tenants making my job ten times more overwhelming and harder.

Later, that afternoon, my father kept saying he wanted to go home. He wanted to see Mama and Papa and find out how they came through our 4.3 and 4.1 earthquakes. He stopped long enough to eat. However, after lunch he started talking about going home. Finally, he took a nap.

The next day, he started talking about going home and seeing Mama and Papa. He even walked around the apartment and figured out how to get out. He walked out onto the porch but he felt cold. I opened the door to follow him and he was ready to come inside, at least for the moment. He eventually decided to go outside in the daylight and the sunshine.

Dad slept most of the day, but we went grocery shopping. Somebody backed into me, the store forgot an item, and I forgot something that I needed.

We came home. He wanted something to eat and then he did not want to eat. He kept calling me to help this guy and give him some money. I am not sure to whom he kept referring but I had a feeling the guy did not exist. I tried to get some work done but I found it quite difficult. He finally fell asleep.

The next day, my father must have been lonely. He wanted to walk over to see me while I was on the computer. He kept asking "Where is Eden?" I had to tell him it was me. Every so often, I would say hi and walk over to him and keep him company for a few minutes.

I do not know if my father is dreaming when he exhibits the following behavior but there have been times at 4:00a.m. that he has yelled "Help" and then thrown his blankets on the floor. He does this several times a night. I have gone over to him to see what is the matter and all he can say is, "Put it together." I do not have a clue to what that relates.

I learned that apparently my father's morning behaviors are commonplace. However, it is just so sad and weird to see and experience these episodes.

I realize symptoms and behaviors can be unique. However, it would be nicer if someone had prepared me a little better for the task and job I have chosen.

Today, as daylight began to wane, my father became more restless. He kept telling me he did not have a room or a place to sleep. He kept asking me, "Where is my room?" Then, he kept asking for the address. I gave it to him. It continued for awhile. I am guessing that part of this confusion regarding his room is because of having to move. We went from a two bedroom to a one bedroom. The move had to be difficult on him. I am still very angry at my former landlord and it will be a long time before I will be able to forgive him.

He told me he felt hungry. I made something to eat. As soon as he finished eating, he started yelling "Help, help" and asking about the address. He did not want to go over to the address as it might have been too late at night. He did not realize he was at the address.

He sounded so sad and depressed. I almost cried. I told him that I loved him and that I would take care of him.

Eventually, he stopped. I love my father dearly but that night, as at other times, he drove me cuckoo.

My father did okay until the sun set and it became dark outside. He took a nap. The nap allowed me to work on the computer and start cleaning the kitchen. Then, my father woke up from his nap. I lost my peace and quiet.

My father must have walked into the kitchen, at the very least, six times for hugs and to see if he could help.

I think he felt lonely and wanted to be needed. I told him I loved him and that he could help by sitting down on the couch. He did but he could not sit without moving. He kept walking into the kitchen.

I finished cleaning the kitchen. The clock read 2:45a.m. by the time I got into bed. I woke up about 8:15a.m.

Later, approximately 7:40p.m., my father became confused regarding his sleeping arrangements. He asked me several times where was his room and where he should sleep. I guessed what he was feeling and validated it. Soon, he calmed down and went to bed. He awoke briefly to go to the bathroom. After finishing what he needed to accomplish, he again asked, "Where do I sleep?"

I expect this behavior to continue considering we moved from a two bedroom to a one bedroom and I have the bedroom. We had to do it this way due to financial constraints.

This is very difficult and it was so unnecessary.

Recently, I noticed several more changes in my father, one of which is losing the ability to remember words. The trauma associated with moving and his medical problems is taking a toll on him. You do not take people with dementia out of a safe routine and move them around as if they were a piece of furniture. It is not good for them. Landlords, especially our former one, do not care. All they care about is money, not people. Well, you cannot have money without people.

Dad had a rough night so I did not get a lot of sleep myself. He kept running back and forth to the bathroom.

He even became confused in daylight. He kept asking me,

"Where do I live? What is the address? Where is my room? Where do I sleep?" He asked the same questions a half dozen times. This is very frustrating for any family caregiver. He also asked me for the very first time, "What is my name?" I said, "David Rosen."

Dad asked questions tonight such as, "Where is my glasses?" He must have asked this question at least four or five times. Each time he asked, his glasses were sitting on his face.

It is difficult to constantly field repetitive questions, deal with difficult behaviors, and watch a loved one fall apart. It takes a lot of patience, love, and self-control. A lot!

People undermine family caregivers when they make stupid remarks because they do not have a clue.

Later, at 6:00p.m., my father began to whine and moan about wanting to go home. For almost four hours all my father said was he wanted to go home, he needed to be home by 8:00p.m., that his mother was waiting for him, and that she expected him to be home. He kept telling me mom was waiting for him and he needed to go home. He thought the apartment was a garage and a junk shop.

His mother passed away almost 36 years ago. I tried to distract him with things he likes, such as hot chocolate, and chocolate cake, etc. It did not work. He became obsessed with wanting to go home to see mom and he would not stray from that path.

He calmed down for awhile but started right back at it. He wanted to go home, mama expected him, and then he thought the apartment was a train station. He also wanted to go out the door. At least, I locked it as I do every night. Locking the door protects him from wandering outside. Dad knew I locked the door. However, he kept asking me at what time I opened the door. He has no conception of time so he would not understand if I told him. He put on his hat and finally laid on the couch for a snooze.

Does anybody want to try fielding such questions as those listed above for more than four hours? Does anybody want to take care of my father and see just how difficult this job is? Then, you might not be so quick to judge a family caregiver.

The next night, dad acted pretty "normal," considering he has dementia, until approximately 10:00p.m. He became restless and wanted to go home. Several times, he tried rising from the sofa and could not. He also tried opening the door but he could not. The door was locked as it usually is at night to prevent night time wandering. After several attempts of trying to open the door, he finally settled down and began to snooze.

Dad became very restless tonight. He paced back and forth several times. He wanted to go home. This time, however, I locked the door. He could not get out. I thought he might become agitated but he did not. I was lucky.

The next night, dad wanted to go home. I told him it would be better if we stayed here because it might rain, it was cold outside, we had everything here, including a lot of love. He dropped it.

Dad woke up. He became restless at 4:30a.m. He was calling "Help" and becoming anxious. He came into my bedroom several times. Then, he went back to sleep and was fine until the evening hours.

I made a few phone calls. He kept calling "Help" for at least an hour. I had to end the conversation to take care of him. Then, I started the computer, trying to get some work accomplished. However, he kept calling me, coming over, and crying "Help, help."

I thought he might be lonely so I asked him if he felt lonely. He told me that he did. I also thought he might need some reassurance so I held his hand, gave him a few hugs, and told him I loved him. This calmed him down. He slept for a little while.

Later, however, he woke up in "difficult behavior mode." I think he was half asleep.

He told me to "put this (a throw blanket) over there on top." I did not know about what he was talking. I asked him where I should put the blanket.

He become agitated, told me he would do it, called me stupid, and told me he would knock off my block.

I moved out of the way. He stood up and walked over into the bathroom carrying the blanket. He did not have it when he walked out of the room.

I walked to the bathroom. He had tossed the blanket on the open toilet seat. Fortunately, the blanket did not fall in the toilet.

I walked back to the living room carrying the blanket. I thought my father would yell at me but he did not. In fact, he did not even remember the "blanket incident."

My father has a wicked sense of humor. However, due to the dementia, I do not know if he is kidding or if he is into his dementia.

I know this incident has to be part and parcel of the disease. My father looked into the bathroom mirror and asked me, "Who is that?"

One day, my father saw his reflection in the bathroom mirror while I helped him dress. I said, "Hi, daddy." Since then, my father has looked into the mirror and said, "Hi, daddy. That is my father" and waves at himself.

Several times, he told me he knew he was the reflection in the mirror or he asked if it was a mirror. Actually, it does not matter if he is joking with me or into his dementia. If it is not attributed to dementia at this time, it could be in the future. People with dementia do not recognize themselves as the disease progresses to its worst symptoms.

I cannot tell you how many times my heart wants to break. This is truly a horrible disease. It robs the people who have it of their whole lives.

Sometimes, my father calls for help and does not realize he is doing it. He told me, "He's calling for help, not me." According to my father, "he" means the other guy who lives here and only exists in my father's mind.

One morning he called for help and began asking, "Where are his clothes?" He did not ask for his own clothes. He asked about the other guy's clothes.

Later, he became very restless. He kept talking about going home to Boston. He wanted to see Mama and Papa. I asked him how he was going to get there. He said he would walk.

As the night progressed, he looked into the mirror and said, "There is grandpa. Hi, grandpa." Then, a few minutes elapsed and he said, "Oh, that is a mirror."

I cannot help but feel sad by the changes and hardship my father is experiencing.

Dad has been very restless. He wanted to go home to see Mama. I had to walk him around outside just to pacify him. After a very short walk, we returned home. He was fine for a few minutes. He started becoming restless. He wanted to go outside to see Mama. He tried to get out of the door but this time he could not open the door.

He wandered around the house, ate some cereal out of the box and dropped it on the floor.

After what seemed like forever, he finally calmed down enough to go to sleep.

The next morning when he woke up, he was soaking wet. He had urinated a lot during the night and even his protective underwear became soaking wet. I took him into the bathroom before we left for my meeting. I had a meeting with Community Services to talk about my "How To Survive Being A Family Caregiver" class. It is not easy being one, and many caregivers, if not all, have a lot of the same issues I keep mentioning.

Later, my dad pooped in his underwear. You expect this from a very young child who is just learning how to potty train. It is heartbreaking and heart wrenching to see this in a parent that you love very much.

The next day, my father woke me at 3:30a.m. for help with the bathroom. Then, later at 6:00a.m., again he thought the apartment was a train station.

Dad became very restless again. He wanted to go home. Fearing that he would push or hit me if I tried to stop him, I walked him outside as he tried to find where the "Rosen's," his mama and papa, lived. He could not find them because they passed away a long time ago.

My father recognized me as his daughter, but he could not recognize home as home.

We walked around the neighborhood. Only one woman asked if we needed help. Every one else ignored us.

We stopped into a restaurant. My father asked if anybody knew the Rosen family or where they lived. I mouthed the word, Alzheimer's. We left. Dad was starting to become agitated, tired, cold, and hungry. However, he would not come home. Where we lived, was not home in his mind.

We walked back to the restaurant. The owner gave him a bowl of soup, several rolls, and a soda. She did not charge me. I also asked a favor. I still could not get him to come home.

I told her to call the Burbank Police and what to say. I basically told her to say that my father had Alzheimer's, he lives with his daughter who is with him, but I could not get him to come home. He recognized me but not home.

As he finished eating, a motor officer arrived. I filled him in and he started walking us home. In the meantime, a patrol car with two officers arrived. They released the motor officer and continued to walk us home. Soon, we arrived. The officers asked if there was anything more they could do to assist. I said, "You could tell him that this is his home and to stay here." The officers obliged. Dad settled down and took a nap on the couch.

My father seems to ask for mama and papa more often now. Sometimes he asks, "Where is Mama?" Other times, he asks about papa. This evening he woke up from his nap saying, "Mama, Mama." The next morning, he did the same thing.

Dad became restless in the morning. He woke me up at 4:00p.m. He wanted to get dressed and go to work.

The next morning, he awoke at 3:30a.m. and wanted to take his blanket, which he thought was something else, to the bathroom. He tried to put it in and or on the toilet. However, I figured out something to say and it worked.

My father wants so much to be independent but he cannot be. This afternoon he went into the kitchen to get cereal. I asked him if he wanted help. He yelled at me. He got cereal all over the floor but worse he put, as those with dementia do, the milk in the freezer instead of the refrigerator.

It is almost two months since we moved. My father is still asking, "Where do I sleep?, Where is my bed?"

Dad became restless yesterday at approximately 4:30p.m. He wanted to "go home." He calmed down for several hours and then became restless again. Fortunately, it rained. The bad weather kept him inside.

During the morning hours, he kept calling, "Hello." He also kept yelling, "Help me, please help me" on and off for approximately two hours. He started this around 3:15a.m. Needless to say, I am tired.

Dad has been seeing water that does not exist and keeps warning me about it. I know it is a hallucination. There seems to be different schools of thought as to whether one should do a reality check or go with the flow.

The next morning, dad woke up at 2:40a.m. He was not agitated but he was very restless, on the verge of becoming angry. He paced back and forth, yelled "Help," got the box of cereal from the refrigerator and took it into the bathroom, leaving a trail of crumbs. He continued to pace and yell help.

I gave him a bowl of cereal and milk. It calmed him down. I cleaned up after him and I finally settled into bed. It was 3:30a.m.

Dad awakened at 3:00a.m. every morning. However, one morning he awoke at 1:30a.m. because he was hungry. I gave him some cereal. He was fine.

However, his restlessness is taking its toll on him. He is so tired, I cannot get him to go to the store. I cannot entice him with the promise of purchasing his favorite cookies.

Inappropriate sexual behaviors are also part and parcel of this disease called vascular dementia. One afternoon out of the clear blue sky he said to me, "Want to suck my prick?" I exclaimed, "Dad!" I reminded him I was his daughter and told him no.

Dad is restless. At 6:00a.m. he was pacing back and forth in my room thinking it was a train station. I also heard him trying to get out of the apartment several times. I could hear the lock jangling as he played with it, trying to open it.

I am just wondering if all of this had to do with going to court on my father's behalf against our former landlord. My father was okay once we arrived at court. I could not help become upset at the Commissioner who presided over small claims court.

We came home. I did a few things around the apartment and then I left to go to work. I worked out in the field but when I returned to the office, I learned that the caregiver called.

She told me that dad was really hyper, tried to get out of the house several times, would not sit still, became agitated, and almost hit her.

I asked to speak to my father. She put him on the phone and I told him to allow her to give him a pill to calm him. After speaking with my father, I authorized her to give him a Depakote.

I returned home at approximately 3:35p.m. Dad was a little calmer. She left almost immediately. I tried to get dad to take a nap. He was still pretty restless but at least he sat down on the couch. Approximately 7:30p.m., he began to become restless and pace back and forth. He wanted money to go home and he rambled. I gave him another Depakote. Eventually he settled down and began to grow calm. This was a very tiring and busy day.

Dad's been pretty restless, probably in part, due to the weather. We cannot even go out. It just continues to rain. He has become a little constipated. He will not let me help him, so I have to do my best. However, I have to tell you, he has been driving me a little cuckoo.

Today, is another long day. It is already after 2:00a.m. He has been in and out of the train station which is, in his mind, in the apartment. I have taken him to the bathroom I do not remember how many times.

I know he is declining. I know just to look at him. He has looked in the mirror and seen everybody else but himself. In his reflection in the mirror, he has waved to his daddy, grandpa, and uncle. At times, he does not believe any more that he is waving to a reflection in a mirror.

It is so sad. I really want to cry. I really hate this disease. People do not have a clue what it means.

Dad was really restless and whiney today. He wanted to go home. He just about drove home. Only kidding, but he really wanted to get out of this apartment. At least, he could not. Instead, somehow I managed to get him bathed and dressed. I cleaned the bathroom.

My father, my aunt, and I went to lunch at the restaurant whose owner treated my father and me with kindness and generosity. The food was good and the portions were big. Considering my father had elimination problems, he did considerably well during and after lunch.

A few days later, dad scared me half to death. I took him to work, the bank, and the grocery store. We got home. He walked up our walkway and reached our two stairs leading into the apartment. He must have grabbed the railing and missed with only a half foot on the step. He fell backward on the concrete and into a bush stump. I called, "Dad, Dad" but he did not respond. His eyes were open but had rolled back. I could only see the whites of his eyes. He sounded like he was breathing funny. I did not believe he was conscious.

I immediately called 911. While I was on the phone with 911, my father started to yell and move. I relayed this to the dispatcher who allowed me to hang up and try to get him to stop thrashing around.

As I was trying to stop my father from thrashing, there were several people around. Only one woman yelled from across the street, "Do you need any help?" I replied, "The paramedics are on their way, maybe you could point them over here." Shortly thereafter, the paramedics arrived.

Two firemen asked me questions while the paramedics took care of him. They cleaned him and took his blood pressure. They helped him inside, walked him around and sat him on the couch.

The paramedics told me he was okay and to watch him and they left.

My father fell mostly in the dirt. Thank goodness he did not fall at my former apartment building. He probably would have died.

However, in spite of him hitting his head and having a bump on it, they did not take him to the hospital. I believe they should have, whether or not his vitals were good. Had they taken him, maybe the trip to the hospital could have prevented certain events from happening just five hours later.

My father misjudged the couch and fell on the blankets on the floor. I tried to get him off the floor but I could not. I placed another call to the paramedics. The same crew came. They checked him again.

My father's vitals were good but he was still stiff and sore from the previous fall. My father was probably scared. They asked me if he normally required as much assistance as they were providing. I told them no. What did they expect? My father is 87 years old and had had a major fall just five hours before.

At any rate, the paramedics told me to take him to the hospital. They said they would take him or I could take him to the HMO. If I had to do it all over again (not that I want to and I hope I do not have to), I would have allowed them to take him to the hospital. After you read the chapter on HMO's, you will understand why I just made this statement.

The paramedics were helpful. However, they did, at one point, open their mouths and insert their feet. It is almost as if they believe nothing happens in nursing homes, day care centers, hospitals, and in the care of professional caregivers. I do not know why they seem to believe this nonsense, but I sure would like to find out.

I sent a letter to the fire department headquarters. I told them to forward my letter onto the appropriate station and captain. I also mentioned for the captain to check my website before he answered and that the paramedics on their off time should volunteer and help someone they think needs help. They may even learn something.

One paramedic said that he knew homes are not good. Another one told me dementia does not get better, it gets worse. Yet, another told me to get around the clock help because I needed it.

Since my father's HMO has not been of any real assistance, I think that considering everything, I am doing a damn good job. I found my father's problem in his breast, not the HMO. Yet, an employee of geriatrics criticized me for my father's loss of six pounds. I will never let so-called helpful advice stick in my brain.

I already know dementia gets worse. I know it is a progressive disease. I also know that there are ups and downs and plateaus where they can hover in for any length of time.

Falls happen everywhere. As one caregiver stated, "The only way to prevent falls is to immobilize them."

My grandmother was in the hospital when she fell out of bed, hit her head and died. My father fell out of his wheelchair in rehabilitation for a broken hip. He fell while in the care of an adult day care center. A caregiver's father fell out of bed in the hospital one night and in the nursing home the next night. One of my former neighbors who used a walker was tripped by a inconsiderate tenant's dog. She fell down and broke her other hip. And last but not least, did our former president not fall down and break his hip? He certainly did. In spite of all the best round the clock help, he still fell down and got hurt. Where was his help?

I think I just proved my point. However, falls happen everywhere and to anybody. An elderly person takes longer to heal after a fall. I fell down and broke the fifth metatarsal bone in my foot. I was 2l. I was in a cast for 6 weeks.

During the last four years, I only remember calling the paramedics three times. One out of the three was totally unrelated to falls. The paramedics have never been so "helpful" until now.

The Assistant Fire Chief called regarding my letter. He felt very concerned and wanted to ask various questions. He asked me if I found their attitudes to be condescending and patronizing. I told him I did. He said he never wanted this to happen to anybody. He said he would handle it at educational and communicative levels and probably would not tell me his findings due to confidentiality matters. I said that was okay.

The Haldol started to wear get out of dad's system. However, as it slowly dissipated, he felt more pain. He started to cry help, yell, and then tell me to leave him alone. I asked him if he wanted to go to the hospital. He said yes. I called 911.

The paramedics arrived on the scene as my father was moaning from the pain. They did not open mouths and insert feet. However, one of the fireman asked me questions so when I turned to answer him, the paramedic said, "Ma'am turn around and look at me." Where is the logic? I needed to be facing the person asking the questions at the time.

They asked if I wanted him to go to the hospital. I said, "Yes." They took him to a local nearby hospital. I met them there.

By the time I arrived at the hospital, talked to the ER personnel, and went into the room, the doctor had already examined him. He was asleep.

Everyone at the hospital was so nice. I only had an issue with one person, the x-ray technician who was a little too aggressive when he tried to turn my father, who winced and moaned in pain. I said, "It hurts." He replied, "I know it hurts, but stop talking and let us get it done."

I really hate these comments. I become angry. There are no valid reasons for the technician's behavior. I reported him by leaving a message on the voice mail for the head of ER. The hospital also has a Service Guarantee and gives patients the right to considerate care. Other than that, as ER's go, it was an okay experience and much better than the HMO.

The doctor ordered x-rays of his lower back, which I believe should have been done on the 28th when I first brought him into the HMO. The hospital also redid the CT scan. There was definitely no bleeding. The test was now deemed conclusive because my father was calm enough to handle it and laid there while the employee ran the test. My father fussed a little but on the whole, he was very cooperative. I wonder if it had anything to do with the difference in the staff's personality!

The hospital discharged him and sent him home in an ambulance because of his condition. He just kept sleeping. In fact, he slept all night and all morning. My poor father. As for me, I did not get a lot of sleep, but I went back to sleep since he was sleeping.

He finally became more awake by Thursday, a good two days after the trip to the local hospital and four days after the HMO gave him too much Haldol. He has been pretty hyper, a little agitated due to the pain, and felt happy after he took the pain pill.

Only time will tell if he will be able to walk more normally than he is doing at this moment. He still wants to fall over and cannot move really well. I have started to squeak quite loudly to the HMO in the hopes they will have a physical therapist come to our apartment.

Dad slept most of the night and day. I surrounded the couch with pillows, blankets, etc. so if he rolled off the couch, he would not get hurt. I snuck out to do grocery shopping as we did not have any orange juice or milk, etc. in the house. I brought home the groceries, put them away and made both of us something to eat.

Dad ate pretty well considering he said he was not that hungry. He also finished a chocolate sundae. He said he felt a little better. He wanted me to help him to the bathroom. I walked him to the bathroom. He stood there holding onto the counter. I guess he is afraid of sitting down and missing the toilet. I stuck the urinal bottle where it belonged and waited. He was pretty wet so I tried to get him to sit down on the toilet. His arms started to shake, then his legs. His knees buckled and down he started. I knew I could not pick him up, so I eased him gently to the bathroom floor and took off his wet underwear. He was conscious.

I called 911 again. The paramedics came out. This time, it was a very different crew. While the paramedics checked him out, one of the crew took down the medical history and another liked the poem, "A Daughter's Lament." He asked when I had lectured at Barnes and Noble on employer/employee relations and customer service. I told him about 5 or 6 years ago.

Anyway, dad checked out okay and we all decided not to go to the hospital. The paramedics said if it happened again to call them and they would take him to the hospital. He is supposed to have an appointment at the Geriatrics department but I do not know how I will transport him. He is not going to make it down the stairs or to the car.

Dad slept last night until about 2:00a.m. However, he went back to sleep and slept most of the day. He got up to eat Chinese food and drink some orange juice. Later, he had some chocolate cake and went back to sleep. A few hours later, he was yelling at me because he did not want to sit down on the toilet. I got him on the toilet, changed his underwear, and brought him back to the couch where he started yelling for his shoes. After not being able to distract him, I gave him his shoes which were lying beside him on the couch. He went back to sleep.

I gave dad a haircut today. He looks a lot better. He even allowed the new aide to partially shave him. She will do the rest a little at a time.

Dad was restless tonight. He kept calling "Help, help," and when I tried to help him, he would holler "Leave me alone." He did this probably about a half dozen times. He also said he had a bundle to give me. The bundle was two blankets that, for some reason, he wanted to give. I love my dad but I found it really difficult to concentrate. Finally, after awhile he fell asleep.

In the meantime, it will be another late night for me. I still have to finish things on the computer, clean the kitchen, and take a shower. I will vacuum tomorrow. I do not think my neighbors would appreciate it if I vacuumed at 1:00a.m.

I never finished the kitchen. I was too tired and had too many things to do. The aide cleaned the kitchen and vacuumed the rest of the rug. She even got down on her knees. Nobody from the agency ever cleaned the kitchen floor even though I have a mop.

Dad does not feel well. Between all the medication, sleeping, and not eating too well, etc., he is constipated. You cannot make dementia patients drink. I know of several family caregivers who have had this problem. For two hours tonight, he was yelling "Help" and then "Leave me alone, help, leave me alone," and so on and so forth. I was trying to work on the computer, but I could not concentrate. He just about drove me cuckoo.

However, I know what caregivers think and how we feel when we think such thoughts. In my case, I wish he would go to sleep for awhile so I could get something accomplished. Yes, there are times when he drives me cuckoo. However, in spite of the disease, I still love my father. I know I would feel very alone and lost if he took that one last very long sleep from which he never awoke.

We finally got through the elimination problem. He finally went. I had to help him since he does not have the muscles to push the waste out and into the toilet. While I was helping to push it out, he hit me several times on the arm. He told me he was going to kill me. Anyway, I managed to get it out. After a while, he felt better and I cried. He told me not to cry because when I cry, he cries. What a rough few days.

Dad's problem turned the other way, at least this morning it did. Then, he slept. He ate a very good dinner but did not eat lunch. He slept. Then, he awoke with a gusto. He barked orders, told me to put his slippers in the corner and then yelled at me when I did not do it, told me to close the various doors several times, etc. He said he did not feel well. I tried to find out what was bothering him. He could not tell me. He also kept calling my name every minute. I lost my patience and yelled at him.

I will be very glad when my professional caregiver comes back tomorrow so I can get out of here.

It was another one of those nights. The professional caregiver was here and she even shaved him. He still has a lot of growth left. Anyway, he was good while she was here but tonight, he tired me out. He just about drove me cuckoo with continuous pleas for help. Then, he threw his blanket on the floor and yelled "Help" so

I could come over and put it back. There were other incidents as well. I stood up and sat down so many times, I began to think I was a yoyo. After about an hour plus of this nonsense, I finally gave him a Depakote to calm him down. Did he? Not for a long time.

I lost my patience. I was trying to work on the computer and go to bed at a decent hour so I could get some sleep. So much for bright ideas. I sat down beside him to tell him he was driving me cuckoo. He said that he was driving himself cuckoo too. Then, he said, "I love you" and he planted a big kiss on me. Afterwards, he told me to leave him alone.

I know he loves me but the dementia does not always allow him to show it, just as I love him, but the disease sometimes makes me lose my patience.

Dad became very agitated during the wee hours of the morning. He tried to choke me. For what happened next, read the chapter on Difficult Behaviors because it fits there better than here.

Dad was restless and agitated last night. He finally fell asleep. He awoke early this morning. It was approximately 6:00a.m. He was soaking wet. He became agitated when I tried to change him. He would not let me. He almost bent my fingers backwards. However, after a lot of I love you messages and a few hugs, dad decided it was okay for me to change him.

He was restless all afternoon. He kept calling me to help him and then told me to leave him alone. This continued for a long time. He finally settled down and had something to eat. He took a nap but when he awoke, he began to yell "Help" and it started all over again. He kept ordering me around. He wanted me to put on his shoes, take them off, put them on, put on his slippers, etc. He started to yell. I came very close to putting him in a home.

I gave him a Depakote to calm him and it worked for a little while. He went back to his nap. However, since he awoke, he has been driving me cuckoo. He asked me if it was raining five times in a minute, questioned me when I told him it was not raining, yelled at me I do not know how many times, called me stupid, dumb, and brainless. Of course, he did even throw in a few kisses here and there.

I am tired and I am out of my medication. I even mailed the prescription while I had three weeks of medication left in the bottle. It sure takes a long time. Anyway, I've got dishes to wash, and I do not know how long it will take me tonight considering he has been yelling on and off all night about things that are not happening such as the rain. I wish I could always figure out what he really wanted and needed.

Dad was very impacted. Stool softeners, prunes, prune juice, an enema, and a suppository did not help. He had trouble eliminating in spite of everything.

I had to physically go in and also had to press on certain areas in order to remove it. My father yelled, called me a few choice names, and told me to go to hell. I cannot blame him. It hurts but I had to do what I had to do.

My father tried to walk through the house half naked. I had to try and get him back on the toilet so I could put on his underwear. He yelled and yelled. I had a feeling someone might call the police.

I barely cleaned him up, walked him back to the couch, and sat him down, when he fell asleep. As soon as he fell asleep, I saw the police walk toward the apartment. I told them I knew why they were here. They explained (which is what I figured) someone called in regarding an elderly person yelling.

I explained that my father has dementia and that he had become impacted, nothing worked, and that I had to go in and help remove it. The police officers peeked inside just to make sure he was okay. Dad was sleeping on the couch. The officers told me, "He is so lucky to have you."

My father will probably yell again and again. The police might show up but at least they know I do not abuse my father.

I gave my father a shower today. He refused to sit on the shower chair. He would not allow me to wash his hair and as soon as he got in the shower, he wanted to get out. I managed to soap up his body and he yelled and hollered while I rinsed him off. Then, he would not let me put new underwear on him and tried to walk out of the bathroom. Somehow, I managed to get him to sit so I could put on his underwear and his shirt.

I guess some elderly folks just do not like taking a shower. I guess babies do not like baths either, but at least a baby is not going to get out of the tub or threaten to kill you because they hate the water.

Anyway, while we were waiting to make sure he was dry, I took care of a few things and then it was time to run some errands. Other caregivers have these concerns so I am going to bring it up. What do you do when you do not have anybody else to watch the care recipient but have to run errands to get protective underwear, cleaning items, food, etc.?

We use our best judgment and pray a lot if we have to run into a store while the care recipient is in the car. Today, there was no problem in the car. I took him into the store to do grocery shopping and he always sits on the chair and waits for me to finish shopping. I would have let him shop with me but I am afraid he may fall down on the floor or some undisciplined child may trip him while playing with a ball he or she does not own. Today, however, he decided to go outside. I found him at the curb. I brought him back. Then, he got up from the chair and wandered about the store. While I checked out, he started walking toward the door, the one farthest from the car, so I went and got him. I had him push the shopping cart. I guess he felt useful and walked with me to where the car was parked. I got him inside and put the groceries in the trunk.

We arrived home, helped him get out, brought him inside, and sat him on the couch. Then, I brought in the groceries and made something to eat.

Later, he started to laugh and got me started and I could not stop. It was the first laugh we shared in a very long time. He just kept cracking jokes. The jokes were not that funny but it was his delivery. Every time I laughed, he started to laugh and I started again and so on until I came back to work on the computer.

I had to bring dad with me today as I did my marketing rounds. He was fine. He became tired later than I thought. He was thirsty. He had part of my drink and all of his. I found soda pop on my car seat where he spilled it. I wiped it up and when I returned home, I sprayed it so hopefully it will not stain. He ate all of his dinner and had several cups of prune juice and his supplement. Then, I put him on the couch and he started to snooze.

Dad was restless this morning. He kept asking about the train and the train station. I finally got those questions squared away when he kept yelling for his shoes. I was afraid he would wake up the neighbors. He went back to sleep. It is now 7:16a.m. Neither one of us slept, although he slept more than me.

Dad slept most of the day. He was restless in the beginning of the evening. He kept calling "Hello, help." and "Help me, please help me."

I cannot tell you how many times I walked back and forth. Every time I approached him, he told me to leave him alone.

I told him he was driving me cuckoo and I loved him. He finally calmed down and fell asleep. He slept until 7:30a.m. the next morning. When he awoke, he spoke nothing but "gibberish" for almost two hours. I helped him to the bathroom, cleaned him, and made his breakfast.

The toilet is still a sore point with him. I do not know why he fights me about helping him sit on the toilet. He becomes so angry that he starts yelling if I try to help him sit. He will not sit. He just wants to go back to the couch rather than sit on the toilet and get changed.

I do not know if it is because he is afraid of missing the seat and falling or because he is forgetting how to sit on the toilet. Rather than admit it, he would rather walk out of the bathroom no matter what is happening.

For example, tonight I tried to sit him down on the toilet. He did not fuss too much but did not sit there very long. I wanted to put a new pair of underwear on him. He got up half naked and tried to walk out of the bathroom. I would not let him. He wanted to choke me but I told him to stop and said, "I love you." Finally, he let me put on his pants. I walked him back to the couch.

I do remind him not to hurt me since I am the only one standing in the way of his placement into a nursing home. If I get hurt, I doubt my brother would take him. Dad would be sent to a nursing home.

Dad became agitated again when I tried to change him this morning. He started to yell at me and made a move toward me as if he was going to choke me. I told him, "I love you," hugged him and again reminded him that if he hurt me, there would be nothing to stop his placement in a nursing home. He calmed down, allowed me to take off his wet underwear, wash him slightly, and pull up the new underwear. However, that is as far as he allowed me to handle him.

Dad was grumpy again when I tried to change him. He yelled, ranted and raved, and wanted to walk around half naked. I threw my arms around him and kept telling him I loved him. He said some horrible things. Finally, he calmed down and sat on the toilet which gave me time to change the pad on the bed, take out clean underwear, etc. Mission accomplished without too many problems. I just wish I could do this without ANY problems. Yeah, right. Who am I kidding?

Dad was very restless later that evening. He cried for "Mama," wanted to go home, asked where he was, almost panicking, and cried "Help me, please help me" every minute. He also would not allow me to change him.

The next morning, I tried to change him and he became agitated and yelled. I found a way to change and calm him. I took him to the couch and sat him down on it. Then, I tried to get him ready to take him with me. He fought me tooth and nail and kept yelling at me. I had no choice but to leave him alone. Fortunately, I found him sleeping in the same place in which I left him.

Dad was pretty grumpy this morning. He would not allow

me to change his underwear. By the time he let me, he was soaked through and through. I tried to put him in the bathtub to give him a shower. He yelled and called me as many names as he possibly could think of at the moment. He stepped into the tub and wanted to get out as soon as he got in. He tried to squeeze my arms. I told him no. He wanted to do something else to me. I told him no. Then, I told him if he stayed in the bathtub and finished his shower, I would give him a piece of chocolate cake. Oh, he still fussed but he calmed down a little. I dried him, put on new underwear, a shirt, and brought him to the kitchen table where he ate the entire piece I put on the table.

Of course, after he finished his shower he was all nice and clean and comfortable. I asked him if the shower was that horrible and he said no. This is his customary response for showers and when I change him. I just changed him and he was starting to get mad. I told him no and to let me do it.

Then, while he was eating some cereal, I said "I bet you feel better now that you are dry and comfortable." He said he felt better. I said "Good and this is why I change you." After he finished his cereal, I brought him to the couch, he sat down, and I covered him with a blanket. He fell asleep again.

Gee, will miracles never cease? Dad allowed me to change him this morning without him yelling at me. He even let me change him later in the afternoon without too much of a fuss.

He slept most of the day so now at 1:39a.m., he is having trouble sleeping. Besides that, he is calling for his "Mama" and asking if his "Mama" is here. My poor father.

I took dad up to Valencia, CA today because I had to take my car to the dealer for its 10 month service. He had a little bit of trouble getting into the shuttle so we could go to the mall to get something to eat. We ate lunch. I bought him a cookie and he sat still long enough for me to virtually run through the mall.

As the time for the pick-up deadline approached, I called for the shuttle to come back for us. It was so beautiful outside we waited on the bench for the driver. Dad had a little trouble getting into the van. He became tired and more grumpy. I managed to curtail some of the "grumpies" and we went back to the dealership. I helped dad into the car and he was becoming more than a little grumpy. I managed to put a stop to the negative behavior without a lot of problems and we headed for home.

He felt tired but he did not really take a nap. Later, I gave him some cake and he tried dozing off again, only to keep calling "Help" and "Help me" every half of a second, at least that is what it seemed. He had a little bit of food and settled down to go to sleep.

Although he had a small "fit" while I changed him, he actually let me do so without screaming and when he started to get a little agitated, I reminded him he would feel better and that I was almost finished.

All in all, he did very well considering how tired he became. However, some days are better than others and today was one of the better ones.

He awoke very early this morning. He was talking "gibberish" and when I walked toward him, he asked, "Who are you?" I told him, "Your daughter." He seemed to understand and went back to sleep.

We did not have a problem with elimination this time. The bran cereal, the prunes and prune juice must be helping. It took two trips but it worked. He even let me change him this morning.

However, by tonight, he was wet and he would not allow me to change him. I hate it when he is stubborn. Nevertheless, he does not know that I am doing this for his own good. I am going to try again.

Tonight, he also called several times for his "Mama" because he thought it was raining on him. After awhile, he knew it was not raining and that it was an hallucination.

Today, I tried to get him out of the house to come with me for my hair appointment. He just did not want to go. He kept telling me he was tired and to leave him alone. I had to call and cancel again. I changed the appointment to Friday and I hope that I can take him to the beauty shop. I really need to get my "mop" cut.

Later, in the evening, he kept yelling "Help, please help me." He would yell this every half a minute; I could not help the fact that he drove me cuckoo. He wanted his shoes. He kept yelling for his shoes. He wanted his shoes so he could go outside. I told him several times that it was too dark outside for him to go out. He finally got the message. Then, after he calmed down about the shoes, he kept yelling help because he wanted to eat something.

I am hoping to run errands tomorrow and get him out of the house with me.

Being a caregiver is not for the squeamish. As dad and I were just about to get in the car and run my errands, he said he had a package and started to pull down his pants. I looked, I saw, I said "Not here" and then we immediately headed for the bathroom. At least, he did not have any problems. It may not be easy cleaning a child after he or she goes to the bathroom, but cleaning a parent is 100 times more difficult and it is heartbreaking to see this.

Once I accomplished the job and got him dressed, we headed for a copy place, the jewelry store for a watch battery, the local paper's office, the mall so I could get my "Do Managers" poster framed, stopped for lunch, and went to several grocery stores. I also managed to stop at one of the card shops to talk to them about the picture cards and check out one of the greeting card company's cards. By the time I hit the grocery stores, dad was getting pretty grumpy and tired. I told him to stop the "grumpies" and that I would put him down for a nap when we got home.

We finally returned home four hours later. Dad was tired. He took a nap and woke up to have a piece of cake and something to drink and then took another nap. He woke up yelling "Help, hello, where are my shoes?," etc. for probably about an hour. I guess I overwhelmed him.

Yesterday, April 21, 2001, was a horrible day. I took dad to the beauty shop with me. He was fine when we walked into the shop. However, after a while, he became very confused. He kept asking, "Where is my daughter?"

If that was not enough, my now former hairdresser made me

very angry. She looked at my hair and said, "With all of your problems, you should let your hair go natural." I told her never. She said she was just asking. Sure, she was asking about something that was not any of her business.

I do not have problems. I have responsibilities. I felt angry. I spoke to several social workers who validated me on the points listed below and above.

Then, the hairdresser, who is in the middle of working on my hair said, "You know we do not take credit cards." I said, "You do not?" She emphatically stated she told me that she made it very clear to all of her customers they only take checks and cash.

I said she did not tell me. I do not remember. I have had too many more important things on my mind. She was my hairdresser for 22 years. One would think she would have trusted me to send her the check. I told her that I would mail the check to her.

Her next comment was also sarcastic. She said, "You realize this is coming out of my pocket." I reiterated that I would send a check. She became more sarcastic and said, "I guess you are getting your hair done for free."

I flatly told her that I was tired (which means I am angry) of getting lectures every time I came in for an appointment and that maybe we should part company after the appointment.

We caregivers can only take so much. I refused to put up with her negative interpersonal skills any longer. I put up with it for 22 years only because she was the only one who could do my hair, so I thought.

She told me that she felt hurt and angry by what I said. What about my feelings? She does not have a clue that her comments are vicious and are definitely not customer service oriented. After a 22 year customer relationship, she inferred that she could not trust me and that I was squelching on my debt.

In customer service, you do not blame the customer or become sarcastic. She also said, "You need to realize . . ." (she did not finish her sentence) because I told her that she needed to realize and I did not get to finish mine. She told me that was enough. She basically told me to be quiet.

Then, she told me she would not cut my hair and to go somewhere else. In the meantime, as if I did not have enough to handle, my father became more confused. He continued to ask for his daughter.

I put him in the car and we headed for home. On the way, I stopped at the place she recommended and had my hair cut.

By the time I was ready to leave, my father became even more confused. He did not know that I was his daughter. He did not want to go out and eat with me and he did not want to leave the shop. Finally, after approximately 15 minutes, we left to go home.

He wanted to eat so we stopped for pizza. He loves pizza. Then, we ran errands and came home. Dad felt very tired and on overdrive. He slept for a little while and then called "Help" every second.

Dad continued to fight on and off regarding changing him. Sometimes he will let me and other times he will not.

Dad's days and nights are reversed. He sleeps during the day and is awake most of the night. I try to get him up, awake, and busy during the day so he will sleep during the night. Sometimes, it is just too difficult and he just wants to sleep.

This morning, dad awoke at approximately 8:00a.m. crying, "Mama, Mama, where is Mama?" He did this for several minutes.

I approached him and said, "Mama's not here but I am and I love you and I will take care of you." He said, "Good" and calmed down when I made that statement. Telling someone you love him or her is a very powerful statement. While it might be difficult for some people to express their emotions on such a heart-felt level, it does work.

A few minutes later, my dad's eyes started to water and he almost began to cry. I asked him why was he crying and he told me he did not know. I kissed him several times and said, "I wuv (I spelled it like this for a reason) you" and gave him a hug. He stopped and went back to sleep and so did I.

Later, I told him it was time to take a shower. He slept most of the day and did not want to shower. This is very common among dementia patients. Finally, at 3:40p.m., I took him to the bathroom. I got him into the shower. He screamed and yelled from the moment he got into the tub that the water was too hot, that he wanted to get out and to leave him alone. Somehow, we managed to get through it.

I made him something to eat and then took him back to the couch. He plopped on the couch and fell asleep. Now that he is awake, he is yelling "Help" and "Hello." Another evening in the life of a caregiver and care recipient.

The local paper interviewed me and sent a photographer to take pictures of me and dad. I hope the story is well written and I am not disappointed.

After the interview, dad pooped. I had to clean him and get him ready for the photographer. He was so adamant about my not changing him and wanted to pull up the dirty underwear and wear it. After he screamed and yelled a little bit, I managed to take off the dirty underwear and wash him. He still had a small fit even though I was doing it for his own good.

The photo shoot went as expected. Dad hammed it up for the camera. He had a lot of fun. I am glad, as I was just a little nervous about it.

Dad slept most of the day and as usual this evening started yelling "Help, help me, please help me." I cannot concentrate when he constantly yells help.

The story came out today. The reporter did a very nice job. I wrote him a thank you note on a "Dad With Friends: Give Me Some Of The Lovin'" card.

I went to bed at about 4:30a.m. Dad woke me up this morning about 7:00a.m. He was yelling for "Mama." I jumped out of bed and told him Mama was not here, I was and I loved him. He calmed down but then he started yelling "Help, help." He was tired so that did not last very long. He went back to sleep and so did I. I am surprised I am still awake. It is now 12:30a.m. of the following day.

However, I did not get a lot of computer work accomplished. Dad started crying "Help me, help, please help, help," etc. approximately at 5:00p.m. It continued until 9:45p.m. It just about drove me cuckoo especially since I am nursing a sore muscle in my mouth and what might be an infection on the backside of the earlobe.

Later in the evening, dad went to sit on the couch, missed it and landed on the floor. He was not hurt. He had not listened to me regarding the right way to sit down. I could not help him get up and he was not hurt so I did not think it was necessary to call 911. I searched for a neighbor and found one. He came over and the two of us lifted dad off of the floor. I then gave directions to my father on how to sit on the couch and this time he listened.

The next day, he slept most of the day. In the evening he became restless and started calling "Help." At least, it was not as bad as the previous day. I knew dad needed to be changed so I bribed him. I told him if he let me change him, I would give him a piece of chocolate cake. Lo and behold I did not have any problems and I gave him the cake. He loves chocolate. Unfortunately, I too have a weakness for chocolate.

I still have yet to give him his shower. I will have to do it tomorrow morning. I am also going to try and get him to the barber tomorrow for a shave. I hope he will go. He is starting to look as if he is a "mountain man" who lives in the forest and never had a shave.

I gave dad his shower this morning. As usual, he started to yell as soon as he got into the bathtub. I washed him really quick and tried to help him out as soon as possible so he would not yell anymore. I managed to quiet him by saying, "No, no screaming!" He yelled while I tried to dry him and put a new pair of underwear on him.

He ate breakfast and went back to sit on the couch. I wanted to take him to the barber but he did not want to go. I hope I can convince him. Anyway, about 5:00p.m., I received a phone call and guess what? Dad could not wait to start calling "Help" and yelling. He finally calmed down until about 8:00p.m. when he started yelling "Help, help, please help me, Eden, Eden," etc. He continued this for over two hours.

He told me that I was driving him cuckoo. Actually, as it turns out, he was driving me cuckoo. He needed to go to the bathroom. I took him and after he went to the bathroom, I began to change him. He started to scream and then called me a "Bitch." I took him back to the couch where he finally fell asleep. I hope he sleeps all night so I can sleep. I still need to clean the bathroom, take a shower, and put the laundry away. It is 12:40a.m. Besides that, the nerve and the muscle in my mouth is back at it again. I had to take a pain pill.

Tomorrow will be my first day of respite since April 3, 2001. I am going to run some errands, maybe watch "Burbank On Parade," go to a nearby park to see the arts and crafts show, and then meet a friend for a late brunch. I do not have to return until 6:00p.m.

I went to buy dish soap and barely returned home before the parade started. Then, I walked to the post office and the copy place to run some color copies. I walked home. I walked around the corner to the park for the arts and crafts show. I found some hand painted pictures that would go very well in the bathroom and came home to get my checkbook. I told the artist about my situation and she gave me a 20% discount. I thought that was very gracious of her. She did not have to give me anything.

I took off for my friend's for brunch. Great brunch. There were cold cuts, fruit, crackers, spread, dip, veggies, and wine. I could not believe how fast the 3 1/2 hours flew by and it was soon time to go home. I returned home a little late.

Dad started calling "Help" and "Help me." However, it was not as bad as the previous days. I helped him go to the bathroom which he needed to do, but he would not allow me to clean him.

He wanted to leave the bathroom immediately after he relieved himself.

Later, he asked where was mama, and mentioned the names of two of his brothers. Two of his brothers are deceased. I do not know about his sister and his younger brother. We lost touch with his family.

Dad did not want to be changed this morning but I managed to change him. He tried walking out of the bathroom before I got his new underwear on him. He hates the bathroom.

Later, dad asked me what I was doing several times. If I opened a box, he asked "What are you doing?" If I stood in front of the television set, he asked "What are you doing?" I think you see where I am going with this. Each time, I told him what I was doing until he got tired and moved onto something new.

I took dad to the barber today. He had so much growth on his face, he was starting to look like I had not shaved him in a month. Anyway, it was worth the $12.00 to have it done by a professional. I just hope dad will allow me to keep it up. I have to admit my father fussed while being shaved but I will also say that in spite of fussing and the dementia, he handled it very well. The barber even put a warm towel over dad's growth to soften it. Dad handled it as if he was a trooper. I rewarded him with two chocolate chip cookies.

It is really difficult dealing with an 87 year-old parent who is stubborn, agitated, and not fully cognizant. It is more difficult than dealing with a child. While I do not have children, I worked in pre-school, day care, and in my psychology professor's school over a five year period. Plus, I baby-sat for over eight years. I took care of infants, toddlers, kindergarteners, pre-teens, and teenagers. I saw a lot of games the children played. I know children can be a handful, but taking care of a parent who exhibits childish behavior is a whole different ball game.

Now on to Chapter Two—Dealing With Difficult Behaviors

CHAPTER TWO

DEALING WITH DIFFICULT BEHAVIORS

My father's difficult behaviors can be caused by health issues; i.e., constipation, the fatigue that comes with chronic lymphocytic leukemia, pain, etc. Difficult behaviors can also be caused by caregiver impatience and lack of training.

As you may remember from my original book, my father had breast cancer surgery on November 22, 2000. In the ensuing weeks after surgery, my father exhibited aggressive behavior toward me. I attribute that to the pain.

On the evening of December 1, 2000, he felt very anxious and wanted to "go home." He kept trying to leave the apartment. Finally he walked outside. I followed.

I told him he needed his jacket. He came with me. I tried to distract him. It did not work and he left the apartment again. As I tried to stop him from leaving the building, he yelled, "Leave me alone." He grabbed my face, arm and fingers. I did not know if he would have broken my fingers. I asked him why he felt so angry with me. I validated his feelings and I responded to the emotion behind the aggressive behavior. Once I did that, I told him to stop because he was hurting me. He stopped. I took him for a short walk around the area on the pretext I was walking him home.

I had to walk him several times. Sometimes it works; other times it does not. At night or when it is raining, I can usually talk him out of it. I tell him I love him, I will take care of him, that it is raining, and that he should stay overnight. More times than not, it works. However, I occasionally have to repeat myself before it sinks inside his brain.

On December 4, 2000, he had an appointment at his HMO. As I helped him out of the car, he called me a "prick." This is also part of the disease. They lose so much. They swear and say or do things that are not sexually appropriate, to name just of a few behaviors they exhibit.

On December 5, 2000, I awoke at 3:25a.m to find my father rummaging through his drawers looking for his socks. He put his pants on backwards. He also had put on his hat. Since they do not have the capability to tell time, I told him it was still nighttime and to go back to bed. This was the wrong thing to say. He said, "Who made you Captain of the Ship? Leave me alone."

I told him I needed my sleep and that I would end up in the hospital. I pouted and pretended to cry. He said, "Honey do not cry, please do not cry. If you cry, I cry." He asked me what he needed to do. I told him to go to bed and off he went.

Approximately a half-hour later, he awoke. He said, "Hello, hello." He wanted to eat. He was adamant. I gave him a supplement to drink and a small piece of chocolate cake. As he drank, he started to sing. Finally, he stopped and as soon as he finished eating, he went back to bed.

It is 4:35a.m. He is snoring and I cannot sleep. I decided to write this portion of the book. Once I wrote everything down, I was able to drift off to sleep. Writing is good therapy because it releases pent-up emotions and feelings.

Later, my father was in the bathroom going on the floor. At the same time, he became very adamant about taking off his pants and protective underwear. I could not take off the garments while he stood. I told him to sit on the toilet so I could take off his clothes. He complied but not before he called me a bitch.

I started to pout and cry. Within a few minutes, he said, "Honey do not cry. Please do not cry. When you cry, I cry."

A few minutes later, he was in a "lustful" mood. He kept trying to hug and kiss me. Then, he asked me to hold his "cock." I said, "Dad" and eventually I brought him back to the reality of the present and that he is my father.

Inappropriate sexual behaviors are part and parcel of the disease. Does anybody still think that this is like raising a child?

One day, I returned from the laundry room. I heard my father calling, "Help, help." He did not need any help. He wanted to bring Mama a glass of water. As you may or may not remember, Mama only exists in my father's mind. However, my father thought Mama was going to die due to the lack of water. He called me a "murdering bitch."

Several times, my father did not allow me to undress him before putting him to bed. He started to become agitated. There were times I let him go to bed wearing his clothes. At l:00a.m., I did not want to start an argument.

Numerous times, my father became agitated by the unprofessional behavior of an aide and started to yell. I had to calm him.

Today, my father wanted to "go home." He kept pressuring me to take him home. He wanted to go home to Mama. He misses Mama very much. Going home can mean returning to a happier time in life.

It is December 2l, 2000. It is l0:40p.m. My father is in bed yelling for his shoes. I told him I had his shoes and asked him where he was going. I guess I said the wrong thing. He called me a dummy and stupid. Fifteen minutes later he told me to put on a light. I did. I asked him if he felt afraid of the dark. He said, "Yes." He also called me sweetheart and gave me a lot of kisses.

Unfortunately, this is the nature of the disease. This is not an easy disease with which to live. It is difficult on both caregiver and care recipient.

I knew my father would experience problems adjusting to the new apartment. He became obsessed with his belief that our new apartment was a theatre. He kept asking me if the people left the theatre. He wanted to find someone he knew from Boston. He wanted to walk around to see if he could see this person. We walked to my bedroom and then the bathroom. Walking seemed to settle my father a little. However, he continually referred to our apartment as a theatre for ten to fifteen minutes.

Besides the theatre, he yelled for someone to close the door. I closed the door way before he yelled. If that was not enough, he kept asking for "Papa, Where is Papa?" I told him he was the Papa. Tonight, for some reason this worked. I did not lie. He is my Papa. However, I think he was referring to his Papa, who had passed away approximately 72 years ago.

While the above examples are probably more annoying than difficult, they are heartbreaking. It is very difficult to watch someone you have loved all your life be reduced to crying for his Mama, his Papa, yelling help every two minutes, etc.

As I fixed the apartment, I must have awakened my father. Dad became very agitated and got out of bed. He started to go into the kitchen clutching at his pants. I knew he had to go to the bathroom. However, he became frustrated, kept yelling "Leave me alone," and went to the couch and sat down. I returned to the task on which I was working.

I know parents fight with their children regarding bath time. However, have you ever tried giving an elderly person with dementia a shower? My father moaned, groaned, and yelled. He drove me cuckoo. Elderly people have thin skin. Hot and cold affects them.

My father told me the water felt hot, then cold, hot, cold, etc. Eventually, we ended the shower session and my father calmed down.

My father can be so "cute" and five minutes later become very agitated. One night, he did not want me to change him or get him ready for bed. He yelled, pushed me, and threatened to kill me. I stayed out of his reach. However, at one point he grabbed my shirt and pulled me. I threatened to call the police if he did not let go of the shirt. Immediately, he stopped holding on to the shirt.

I went away, took my night-time shower and cried my eyes out. He came into the bathroom. I told him to go away. He did. I was still crying when I came out of the shower. I put on my nightgown and went to face my father. I could not stop crying. By this time, as is usually the case, the difficult behavior disappeared. My father hugged me and kept repeating, "Please do not cry. Do not cry." Eventually, I stopped and he allowed me to change him. Peace had been restored to the household.

People are totally clueless when it comes to this disease and the heartbreaking effects it has on family caregivers and family members.

There will be more examples in this chapter. Difficult behaviors come and disappear very fast.

Several days later, my father became rather grumpy. He kept asking me "What is wrong?" I repeatedly told him nothing was wrong and that I loved him. This did not pacify him. Finally, he went back to sleep. We both had a rough night.

At one time, he said, "Who are you?" I said, "Daddy, I am your daughter, Eden." I think he understood. He said, "Hi daughter" but then he called me by my brother's name three times.

He took a nap and when he woke up he felt confused but did not manifest any difficult behaviors.

Dad is being difficult again. He told me he was going to break my hand. He squeezed it quite hard. He threatened to knock off my block and made a fist.

Previously, I tried to assist him with his bathroom needs but he became very agitated. He yelled at me to go away and leave him alone. Then, he kept hollering "Help." Every minute, he would yell, "Help."

I stayed up pretty late. I could not get anything accomplished. I had to stop and go take care of him every time he yelled "Help" to make sure he felt okay. Later, my father became agitated but settled down quickly. He allowed me to give him a bath. Still later, he needed to be changed. However, he became very agitated and would not let me change him. Once he calmed down, I told him I wanted to change him so he would feel more comfortable. He seemed to understand and drifted off to sleep.

It is now the first week of January. My father yelled "Help." I walked over to him to take care of him. He needed to go to the bathroom. I helped him into the bathroom and caught him so he could pee into the urinal. If I do not help him, he pees on the floor. He became very angry with me, pushed me and told me to leave him alone. I told him he was hurting me and to stop. He stopped.

We started the second week of January. My father became very grumpy. He yelled and told me to leave him alone. However, he also told me to prepare a particular shipment to La Porte, Indiana. We do not know anyone in Indiana. He became obsessed with the shipment. After he yelled at me several times and got on my case several times, I yelled back.

What can I say? Being a family caregiver is not easy.

Most of my father's difficult behaviors manifest themselves during the toileting process. I have problems cleaning him and assisting him in the bathroom even when he knows who I am. I think it is because he is a very proud man and he knows he is losing his independence. I know this is difficult for him. I can see it in his behavior. He understands what is happening to him at some level.

Notice, I said most of my father's difficult behaviors manifest themselves during toileting. However, not all of them.

My father's difficult behaviors are hard on me. There are no advanced warnings, at least in my father's case. He can erupt just like an earthquake.

I was sitting and watching TV, minding my own business. My father yelled at me to get out. He kept yelling at me to get out and not come back.

At one point, I asked him why he was so angry at me. He told me I was no good and he wanted me out of the apartment.

I prepared my dinner. As I made dinner, he told me to get out. He also told me that he was calling the police and have me arrested.

I finished preparing my dinner and ate it. By the time I finished eating, my father's behavior returned to wanting to give me love.

Later, he asked me where the fellow went. He said the fellow ate dinner and left. He did not know who was the fellow.

I had my suspicions my father did not recognize me. However, I did not realize to what extent. Telling him that I was his daughter did not register. To him, I was the fellow he told to get out and on whom he wanted to call the police.

There is something about the bathroom and changing him that upsets him. If I could definitely put my finger on it, things would be easier. He became quite agitated when I told him I was going to change him so he would feel dry and comfortable. He yelled, grabbed my face, squeezed it, and grabbed my hand and squeezed that as well. He told me he would kill me. I told him to stop. I had to threaten to call the police but he stopped.

I do not hate my father. He does not know what he is doing. I hate the disease. Anyway, a few minutes later, he came back to reality. He told me to come and sit down. I asked him if I could change him. He told me I could change him and he would not punch me. I changed him and things were fine. He told me to sit down, and give him a kiss and a hug. He also said that he loved me. I almost cried.

I had a feeling something might be bothering my father when I made lunch and he told me it was garbage and he would not eat it. I made him something else a little later. He complained about it but at least he ate it.

Dad did not know who I was. He ordered me out of the house, to never come back, and called me a phony. After awhile, I walked outside and hid by the garage to regain my composure and for him to return to reality. By the time I returned, my father was asking for help and looking for me. However, it did not stop me crying. He gave me a hug and told me to stop crying.

Sometimes it has been my experience, in order to prevent a catastrophic reaction, one has to leave the area rather than confront. The behavior does not last.

Later, my father yelled at me but he became aware of what he did and apologized for being so boisterous.

Still later, he yelled at me again to turn off the lights and said that I was responsible for his lack of sleep. I doubt that. However, I could not go to sleep because I could hear my upstairs neighbors' television in my bedroom. He yelled at me to get out of the kitchen. He tested my patience to the max. Patience lost. I even started to cry. He kept telling me, "Do not cry. When you cry, I cry." I still cried. I finally stopped, but it took me awhile. Every time he told me not to cry, I cried.

The irony of the situation is that he never remembered yelling at me. They usually do not remember their extreme behavior. My father is not any different as shown by the above examples.

Today, I tried to get him into the shower, but he did not want to go. He said he felt tired. I let him snooze. I was minding my own business writing some letters while he slept. He woke up periodically because he thought something was burning on the stove. I told him no. He dozed and woke up a few minutes later to ask me the same question. I told him everything was okay.

However, he followed my every move with his eyes. I sat down to write and he just started yelling at me. He yelled, "Get out of here. Leave me alone. Get out of here or I will throw you out." Then, he said, "Son of a Bitch" as he tried to get off the couch. I said, "Okay, I am getting out of here," took my items and hid in my bedroom. I wonder, as I write this, how long he will take to change.

I came out of the bedroom walking on eggshells. He was still sleeping. He woke up hungry but he was fine. Again, he did not remember yelling at me.

He was restless all evening and all night. He kept telling me he wanted to go home. He also kept looking at my pictures and posters on the wall and saying, "That is my daughter, Eden." However, when I asked him who I was, he could not answer. He did not know.

Later that night, he really became restless, pacing back and forth, moaning and groaning how he wanted to go home. I tried saying that I loved him and I would take care of him and that we had everything here for him. It helped for awhile.

Then, about 10:50p.m., he walked out the front door. I tried to distract and stop him from leaving. He gave me his arm in my neck, pushed me, and walked out the door. I fell backwards, slid over the table, and onto the floor crying. He said, "I am sorry, good-bye," and he walked out the front door.

By the time I got up off the floor and pulled myself together, I went out to look for him. He was two blocks down. They can sure move when they are in "wandering mode." As I walked down the street toward him, I was still crying. I caught up with him. He asked me what was wrong. I told him what he did while the tears just streamed down my face. He kept apologizing and telling me not to cry.

As we walked back, my father's leg started to give way but we made it. He wanted to go the other way, but he walked me home all while apologizing for pushing me.

I am still very teary and a little stiff.

The next day, I went to my HMO to make sure I did not break anything. I had a very slight sprain in my wrist, pulled muscles in my back near my shoulder blade, and a few bruised ribs. The nurse gave me a rib belt to wear for a week and scheduled a follow-up visit.

I returned to my HMO for a follow-up visit. The doctor told me I would feel sore for approximately three weeks. She prescribed 800mg. of Motrin 3 times a day. That is a lot. You should see the size of these pills. They are huge.

Understanding someone with dementia is a very difficult task for a family caregiver. As dementia and Alzheimer's recipients lose their ability to form words, speak, and or communicate clearly, it becomes more difficult to understand them.

For example, my father yelled at me to go to bed. I was trying to accomplish some work on the computer. I began to lose my patience. There are times I do not have much patience left in my being.

Anyway, my father began to yell at me, "Go to bed." He must have said this six or more times. After the sixth time, I gave up counting. At one point, he told me he was going to kill me this week and to go to bed.

All of a sudden, an idea popped into my brain. I lowered my voice and said, "Are you yelling at me to go to bed because you want to go to bed and I am disturbing you?" That was the magic question. He answered, "Yes." I turned one of the lights out, covered him with a blanket, and he went to sleep.

The day we went out to the HMO, he kept yelling at me to shut off the light and go to sleep. Finally, I made a deal with him to give me a half-hour more computer time.

I could not handle anymore (read the chapter on in-home agencies because they really made me angry). I started to cry. My father told me not to cry but I could not stop.

I find it very difficult understanding, what I call "dementia-ese." Not understanding it can cause a lot of problems.

I still do not think that my father's difficult behaviors are totally caused by the progression of the disease. It does not matter whether or not he thinks I am a stranger or his daughter. I can see his reaction to the way I respond to him as proven by the incident in which he pushed me.

If anybody thinks this is still like raising a child, even a very young one, then you really are clueless. It is time for education.

Dad is constipated and he is miserable. I do not know how he can be constipated by the amount I helped push out.

Anyway, I tried to take him to the bathroom. We passed my bedroom on the way. He wanted to lay down in my bed. I told him no. He persisted. I told him no several times but he still persisted. He grabbed my arm, then put his hands around my neck, started to squeeze, and threatened to kill me.

I managed to stop him from choking me. I started to cry and I could not stop. He told me to stop and said, "Please don't cry. Honey, do not cry. When you cry, I cry." However, he still would not allow me to take him back to the bathroom.

I tried to go back to sleep but could not. I finally got into bed at 4:30a.m. It is 3:20a.m. the next morning. I am dozing off and I have to be up relatively early tomorrow.

Today was one of those days. I took him for his follow up visit to the surgeon who did the breast cancer surgery. I parked in the lot and we caught the tram to the entrance. The driver helped me walk him toward the door. We managed to get him upstairs and checked in. We got him through his appointment and I got him back into the car to run errands before going home.

We arrived home. He did not want to get out of the car. Then, he got out of the car and said a number of things I did not understand. I did not know that getting "an attachment" was "dementia-ease" for "I have to go pee." Before I could do anything, he whipped out "Uncle Peter" and urinated in the driveway. Then, he got back into the car.

I tried to get him out of the car but he threw a temper tantrum. He yelled several times. He yelled at me to leave him alone and then he put his thumb on my Adam's apple and pressed. He also threatened to kill me. I told him to stop it, grabbed his hand and said, "I love you." He called me a bitch and a few other choice names. Finally, he calmed down. I got him out of the car, got him into the apartment, placed him on the couch, took off his shoes and let him take a nap before dinner.

I saw a police car drive by. I thought they might stop here since he was yelling, but they just drove down the street.

He is doing better. However, he is tired and he became grumpy and agitated again. He yelled at me over something I could not recognize and called me a "Shtunk," a Yiddish or German word which approximately means stinker.

The next day, the professional caregiver came to take care of dad. I do not know the entire story but she said that he put his hands on her shoulders as if he was going to hug her. Instead, he pushed her backwards. She was trying to change him and clean him and he would not allow her to do it, so he became agitated.

Dad was agitated today. He became impacted again. I gave him prunes, prune juice, bran cereal, supplement, coleslaw, and he still had a heck of a time going to the bathroom. I thought the police might come here again. I had to physically try to relieve some of the pressure in his body. He yelled and even when I did not touch anything, he yelled. He also squeezed my arm to the point he was hurting me. I had to tell him to stop. He called me a "basket," which I assume is dementia-ease for "bastard." He called me a bitch numerous times as well as a stinker. What can I say? Nothing. I know it is the disease talking, not my father.

He's been grumpy and whiney all night. I guess I would be too if I had his problem. He keeps yelling, "Help me" and then, "Leave me alone." It is enough to drive any sane person cuckoo. I would really like to get this problem resolved as soon as possible for both our sakes.

Difficult behaviors are part and parcel of the disease. Sometimes one can distract the care recipient but that does not always work. I found that finding the emotion behind the behavior and validating those emotions helps eradicate difficult behaviors. Of course, since my father and I are still connecting, crying helps alleviate some of his agitation and aggression; at least in my case it works.

Now onto Chapter Three—HMO Issues

CHAPTER THREE

HMO ISSUES

In November 2000, my father had surgery for breast cancer.

On December 4, 2000, the surgeon wanted me to bring my father in for a follow-up visit. A lot of fluid accumulated underneath his arm from the surgery. The surgeon drained 500 cc's of fluid. He said he removed the drain sooner than he wanted. However, he wanted to spare me the hassle of dealing with it. He obviously knew my father would react to it.

The surgeon also left the staples and told me to return in a week. The next appointment was December 14, 2000.

During the visit to the HMO, I took my father to get his flu shot. I asked one of the receptionists where they were giving the shots. She said, "In the other building and the hospital lobby." I ran into another employee and asked her. She told the receptionist to call and double check. It is a good thing she did. We would have gone on a wild goose chase and my father already felt tired. If the receptionist was customer service oriented, she would have called without anyone asking her to double check.

We walked to the next building. My father does not get a lot of exercise. I figured I would tire him out. After a student nurse gave him his shot, another found a wheelchair. He took him outside where we could catch the tram. The driver dropped us off at the car.

I brought my father in to see the surgeon for the follow-up visit. The surgeon drained more fluid from my father's armpit and took out the staples. We were told to return December 22, 2000.

The day of the appointment we received a phone call regarding a cancellation and we rescheduled the appointment for January 2, 2001. On January 2, 2001, the surgeon told me that he discussed my father's treatment with the oncologist/hematologist for the breast cancer. There would not be any treatment for the chronic lymphocytic leukemia but they would prescribe Tamoxifen for the breast cancer. The doctor told us to return in three months.

Today, I received a phone call from the department administrator of the geriatric clinic regarding my follow up concerning the dinner check. (Story in original). She received all of my letters and would track down the check they were supposed to send to reimburse me for my father's dinner in June 2000. I told her if they sent it, I do not remember receiving it. She said she would call accounts payable and get this resolved. So far, I have not received the payment or a call. Membership services authorized it. I wonder if they are stalling.

I called today and left messages for both the administrator of Geriatrics and member services regarding this check that has not arrived as of this writing.

I received a call from both parties. The check is in the mail or should be very soon. The administrator said the check caused her to get gray hairs. I told her that various employees in the department gave me gray hairs. She told me we were even. I told her not by a long shot.

I received the check about 10 days later. Finally!

Today, we saw the hematologist/oncologist for both my father and myself. My father gained weight and the doctor prescribed Nolvadex, generic for Tamoxifen. Tamoxifen is a hormone blocker. Breast cancer is caused by a hormone. In men, the hormone comes from the adrenal glands. In women, the hormone comes from the ovaries.

Anyway, the doctor gave me a compliment. He said I was doing a good job for my father. I try. Lord knows I try. He is the first HMO doctor to ever give me a compliment.

As you have read in the previous chapter, the paramedics suggested that I take my father to the hospital for evaluation. They helped him into the car and off I drove.

What happened at his HMO was a nightmare in itself. Once at the HMO, I was allowed into the ER while the doctor evaluated him. The doctor did not check his eyes to see if his pupils were equal and reactive. He did not perform the "follow the finger" test. Maybe doctors do not do those tests anymore. He ordered blood and urine tests. They did an EKG and a chest x-ray. All the tests came back okay so he was released. He did not order a CT scan. The doctor told me that the head is the hardest part of the body. Oh, please! Does he really think I am stupid? The head might be the hardest part of the body but eventually head injuries, even minor ones, can cause problems.

I have enough stress in my life and they increased it, but that is not unusual. My father does not like hospitals, doctors, etc. One nurse kicked me out because she wanted to draw blood. What did she not want me to see? Did she think I was squeamish? Leaving the room because she needed to draw blood is a bit much. I went to the doctor and told him what she said. The doctor called the nurse and told her to allow me back in because I would be a calming influence on my father, or as the doctor put it, "Let her stay because he is a handful." I had problems but I calmed him down to the best of my abilities. Maybe he would not have been such a handful if they knew how to treat people with dementia. After all, compare the treatment and attitude at the HMO to the one given at the local hospital, with the exception of the X-ray technician.

My father can pick up on the feelings of others, and his regular nurse was way too rough on him. The nurse tried to get him to urinate. My father could not go to the bathroom. The nurse said in front of me, "You need to pee, David. Otherwise we'll have to stick something up your penis to extract the urine and it is not very pleasant." I gave water to my father to drink and he complied. However, he went so much he wet the bed. (If they had given him an enema for his constipation as I requested, they would have gotten the urine out of him a lot faster).

The nurse and another employee changed the bedding. They rolled him over and agitated the hell out of him. He was stiff and sore and they were not gentle.

They did not put anything on the scratches on his lower back. They did not put anything on the sores on his scalp until I mentioned it to the nurse. He only put some antibiotic ointment on it as we were getting ready to leave. We were there until 2:15a.m.

In spite of my father's agitation the nurse wanted to roll him over on his side to pull up his pants. I emphatically said, "Let's not! Stand him up and once he is out of bed, then we will pull up his pants." My father did not yell or holler. Problem resolved.

Now it was time to put dad in the wheelchair and take him to the door so he we could put him in the car. This almost caused WW3. The nurse tried to put him in the wheelchair and grabbed him under the arm and started to pull my father toward him. My father became agitated again. The nurse tried two times. He tried to put him in the chair a third time and I put a stop to it. I told the nurse to back off and that some people just cannot handle dementia patients. Listed below is how I handled my father and the wheelchair situation.

I placed my hands on my father's shoulders. I told him to focus on me. "I know you are afraid of falling. I will not let you. The nurse is holding the chair and I have you. Step back until you feel the chair at the back of your legs and then sit down." My father understood. The problem was resolved. Why do I have to teach nurses how to deal with dementia patients? They are supposed to know how to handle people. This is ridiculous.

I asked for help from the other caregivers, especially those with medical training. The responses included: "What was the doctor thinking? What is up with the medical professionals in your area?" and "Why did they not do a CT scan? They should have done one."

Since the ER personnel also ignored my plea for an enema

and I have a very small bathroom, I took him to the HMO's closest facility for assistance with the enema. I really do not have a place to give him one here. The receptionist told me that they do not give enemas any more but she would find someone.

The receptionist found someone. As if I do not have enough stress in my life, the nurse added to it. After she gave him the enema, he went to the bathroom immediately. When he was finished, she discussed my father's problem in the lobby in front of others. Besides showing such unprofessional behavior, she made suggestions not knowing how my apartment is arranged.

She told me to place my father on our couch and give it to him on the couch. I told her the couch was not near the bathroom and added "You saw how fast he went after you gave it to him. He would never make it to the bathroom." Then, she told me to place him on the floor on the carpeting near the bathroom. What the hell was she thinking? I am going to put an 87 year-old man on the floor? I do not think so! Her last suggestion was that I should do it the way she did it. I told her my bathroom was way too small for two people.

Then, she told me I needed help taking care of him. I asked her in a rather loud voice, "Are you offering to come over and take care of him for free?" She said "No." I told her to not discuss it anymore.

The HMO is supposed to provide a service. Part of that service is helping those people that need help. I really do not care if they are an HMO. Medicare recipients in HMO's are entitled to the same care as an 80/20% Medicare recipient on Medicare.

I complained to the unit manager who left to oversee the laboratory within the same organization but a larger facility. He called to say he felt concerned and that he was forwarding my e-mail to the doctor in charge of the facility.

I heard from the Care Manager in the local HMO facility. She gave me some numbers to call to help me. I did not know there was a Member Ombudsman at the hospital to which the clinic is connected. I will go into greater detail because it took me a few days to call the numbers she gave me.

Now, I know that the HMO does not always follow its policies and procedures that do not allow family members to go into ER with the patient. I know other people who have gone into ER with their loved ones and just a few days before they allowed me to go into ER without any problems.

On Sunday, March 4, 2001, my father and I returned to the HMO's Urgent Care department as per the instructions on the sheet. They sent me back to ER. At least I only had to pay $10.00 and not $20.00.

However, the nightmare continued. An Urgent Care nurse brought him to ER. They took him into ER without me. This nurse, who should not be in ER, told me that I could not go back with my father for 15 minutes. I told her that was not a good idea. I told her that he has dementia and that he would become very agitated if I was not with him. She ignored me and stated that policies and procedures did not allow for "visitors" until the doctor evaluated the patient, a process of about 15 minutes.

I knew that this was not true. I know they bend the rules so I became angry. I told her I was coming back with him. She started to argue with me. She made me angrier. I started to yell. Then, she told me I should not attack her and that she was trying to help me. When will people in the medical field learn that statements such as these tend to escalate situations, not diffuse them? I demanded to see the patient advocate and then told her that if she really wanted to help me she needed to validate how I felt at that moment. She never did and she continued on with her very brusque personality and lack of customer service attitude. She told me they did not have one. Then, she found a supervisor and told me she was a patient advocate. In the meantime, I saw the nurse we had the first time I brought him into ER. He started to ask me what was wrong. I told him he was not touching my father. He asked why, so I told him. I told him he did not know how to deal with dementia patients. I spoke the truth.

By this time, the supervisor arrived and we went into a room to talk. She told me I was very knowledgeable. Gee thanks, but I would rather get the customer service from the employees instead of being yelled at and criticized.

While I was talking to the supervisor, the nurse came in to tell me that she had been looking for me because my father was quite agitated. She asked me to help calm him. However, my father had become so agitated, I could not calm him. Had I been allowed to come inside the ER from the very beginning, I might have been able to calm him as I had on the 28th of February.

The doctor had to give him medication to calm him so that they could do the CT scan. They gave him 1 milligram of Ativan and apparently anywhere from 7.5 to 10 milligrams plus of Haldol. They over medicated him. They sent him home in an ambulance at approximately 9:45p.m. because he would not have been able to get in the car and walk.

The doctor said my father would be drowsy and would sleep all night but that he would be okay by morning. It is now 11:30a.m.. He is still very drowsy and tired. At 1:30a.m. the next morning, he was still sleeping. A lot of the medication is still in his system. Hopefully, it will wear off by late morning.

The discharge notice states, "He will be drowsy tonight." I complained. This is one paragraph from a letter from membership services regarding my complaint: "Your concerns and your father's medical records were reviewed by the appropriate administrator who informed me that your father was very agitated and needed to be sedated so that a CT scan could be done. He was given I.V. medication slowly and the dose was titrated for effect and he was monitored. It was also noted that you were advised that he would be sleepy and drowsy, especially since he is older."

I do not know about you, but how does you were advised that he would be sleepy and drowsy but okay by the morning translate to Thursday evening? This HMO has a bad habit of twisting everything around to fit their screw-ups.

The drug is supposed to be injected into a muscle, not directly into the bloodstream. I do not call 2.5mg every 30-45 minutes for a total of 7.5mg or more "given slowly." However, the most important question I have is why was "No Haldol" not on the computer or in the chart? If not, why not? If so, why didn't the doctor ask me? I told the nurse when my dad had breast cancer surgery that they were not to give him any more Haldol. I saw her write it on his chart.

The HMO has a Service Guarantee dedicated to treating patients and families in a caring, respectful, and dignified manner. I sure wish they would follow it. Here are excerpts from it.

We will: Communicate and act in a professional manner conveying compassion, courtesy, and empathy. Ask questions and listen carefully to your responses so that we can understand your needs. Treat you in accordance with the Patient's Bill of Rights. Strive to resolve problems immediately whenever possible.

Unfortunately, I had to remind certain employees about the ER's own Service Guarantee that, ironically, is hanging on the wall right near the reception area.

I placed another call to dad's primary physician. The doctor returned my call and I told him what happened. I also told him that some of the caregivers who have medical credentials told me that I should take my father to a neurologist. The doctor told me a neurologist would not help as my father has severe dementia. A neurologist would only help someone in the early stages. I find it ironic that because of his age and the dementia they do not want to do cataract surgery, and do not want him to see a neurologist, but they would rather have him fall and chalk it up to the dementia and maybe the medication.

The way some of the employees talk, my father has "one foot in the grave" and is a lost cause. Then, why did the employees tell me he needed surgery if these are his last days?

I spoke to my father's doctor and updated him as to what happened. The doctor agreed that I should wait until the next day to give him the pain medication and to let him sleep it off. He said the scans are normal so he could be just very tired or the disease has progressed. He agreed that a traumatic experience could cause a decline. Maybe, the doctor is finally learning that I do know something. It is about time. However, knowing the HMO, I wonder.

If you will refer to my original book, the adult day care center personnel told me that the incidents in the center were caused by the progression of the disease. If the doctor does not know if certain things are due to the progression of the disease, how could a program director of a day care facility? This is comparing apples to oranges. The doctor has an M.D. degree. The program director, a BSW. Nobody should be making an assumption of any kind.

The next day, I was on the phone almost all afternoon with the HMO trying to resolve these issues. What a waste of my time. I sure wish it would get its act together. I called the patient advocate (member ombudsman) but she was out of the office. She had a referral number to Administration. I called the number and told the person who answered the phone the story. I told her that some of the issues pertained to the other facility but I called because it also pertained to the doctor who worked out of Glendale. I told her what he said about taking my father to a neurologist, which was that the neurologist could not help my father because he had severe dementia. He might have been able to in the beginning stages. Ironically, the HMO never referred me to one in 1997. So what else is new?

The local hospital suggested physical therapy, but nobody at the HMO mentioned it at all. My father is having a lot of trouble walking, as well as standing, and nobody mentions PT. Is this a great HMO or what?

The local hospital told me to call dad's primary physician and request pain pills for the pain in his back. Nobody at the HMO bothered to even say (as if they did not know he was in pain. Please!) as soon as the effects of the medication wear off, you may want to put him on pain pills to ease his suffering.

My next phone call was to the department administrator of social services. However, they would not let me talk to her. The

excuse the employee used is that she is the department administrator and she would just assign it to a social worker. Then, the
employee said, "I will page the social worker for you who handles
the clinic."

I spoke to her. I told her as much of the story I possibly could.
She interrupted me several times to ask my age, my medical condition, etc. Then, she did what the other HMO employees do
when they hear their personnel screwed up. She said to me, "Have
you considered a convalescent hospital (as if I would not have stress
if I placed him) for your father?" She turned it around and laid it
on me. Please! I told her that my father would give up and die,
that he was entitled to the same care that a 80/20% patient on
Medicare should receive, and that I was very tired of reminding
HMO personnel of this fact. She had opened her mouth, inserted
her foot, and I called her on it. She did not say another word
regarding this matter.

After I completed the conversation, I sent her my "Family
Caregivers need recognition, support, and love" article that was
published in my local paper. I sent a copy to the patient advocate.
Who knows? Miracles do happen.

I requested a visit from the Home Health nurse and a physical
therapist because my father has trouble walking. I could not bring
him anywhere. Geriatrics made an appointment toward the end of
the week.

I told the nurse that I would call her the day before to let her
know. However, after what just happened, I called the geriatric
department's voice mail and left a message. I told them what happened and that there was no way I could get my father to his
appointment.

I hope the HMO can resolve this issue since some of this is
their fault. Of course, they will never admit that. The patient advocate and the person to whom I spoke in administration never
returned my call. This is not good service. In fact, this is no service
at all.

As for geriatrics, they still want me to bring my father in on

Thursday. However, in order to do so, I would have to pay for the van ride or transport. Prices range from $40 and up plus mileage. Difficult to pay for when one is on a tight budget. I tore up the list of companies and threw out the garbage. The HMO will have to do better. The social worker called me and said that only dad's primary physician can order an ambulance. If that's the case, how did emergency send him home via ambulance after they overmedicated him? I am sure they did not call his primary doctor at 9:00p.m. However, stranger things have happened.

I e-mailed the social worker stating that since the HMO overmedicated him, the HMO should pay for the van ride. She called me to say that the "ride" was not covered. I said okay. I later e-mailed her and told her the figure in my head that was going to legal was increasing all the time. Here the HMO over-medicated him and they will not cover the van ride. I am not a very happy camper.

Also, the employee from Administration never called me back regarding my complaint or request. This is such great customer service (several people told me I am good when I am sarcastic).

I reported the HMO and several doctors to the California Medical Review Board regarding the overdose of medication, not taking pelvic x-rays or the CT scan, etc. They will look into it. It is a very long process but maybe I will have some answers. I feel very frustrated.

I have written letters to the National Accreditation Quality Association (NCQA) about the HMO, the Department of Managed Care, and my state representatives.

I just want to scream. My father had his geriatric appointment on March 22, 2001. I do not agree with the doctor's assessment that my father shook because he felt weak and he is getting weaker. I truly believe and so do others that he shook the way he did from the overdose of Haldol.

The doctor told me that when people are near the end, they sleep more. This may be true but not necessarily. The Tamoxifen and the Depakote and the overdose of Haldol made him very tired.

Besides that, after I dropped off my father and the aide, I had to run some errands. She fed him and put him on the couch for a nap. I got home, she left, he got up from his nap and started to cry. He felt depressed.

Depression can make the dementia worse and it is not necessarily part and parcel of the dementia. A lot of things can cause depression.

I want the HMO's personnel to start thinking in shades of gray instead of black and white. They have chalked everything up to the disease and they only see him once in three to four months.

I have become very tired of becoming the "walking file cabinet," the "trainer," and being treated as if I do not have an intelligent brain in my head. Many caregivers feel and have been treated the same way. It makes our job as family caregivers more difficult.

The doctor kept verbally throwing things out at me and with the exception of the DNR, did not give me time to think about it. I told her I was overwhelmed. She immediately assumed that I was overwhelmed due to caregiving duties. She told me, "Of course you are; caregiving is very physically and emotionally demanding." DUH! As if I did not know this. However, in this case, I told her that was not what was overwhelming me.

I spoke to her later, and she told me the only reason she ordered the bed was because the professional caregiver I brought with me agreed it was a good idea. At the same time, however, the doctor stated that she believes in the value of family caregivers. Is that why she did not even ask me if I wanted the bed for my father? I had concerns about the bed. I know my father would probably climb over the railings. He did it in rehabilitation and prior to hip surgery at the hospital. Other care recipients have tried to climb over the railings and have gotten hurt. If my father was no longer ambulatory, then the bed, as long as it had full rails, would probably be great but now is not the right time.

She also mentioned that I should start thinking about placing my father and keep it in the back of my mind since the disease gets worse not better. Really? I told her I was not ready to sign my father's death warrant. Nevertheless, I have thought about it since he was first diagnosed almost four years ago.

I just keep on trucking. I think it is also because the HMO's employees kept on me about placing him and telling me how bad of a caregiver I am. I have a feeling there is something subconsciously in my mind that says when they tell you that you cannot handle it, etc,. you show them! I continue to show them!

She also told me that some kind of spot or something showed up on the x-rays he took on February 28, 2001. She reordered the x-ray as a comparison to the one taken in February.

She told me the doctors did not know what it was. They did not know what it was, did nothing, never bothered to tell me. Is this great or what? Even if they suspected or did not suspect lung cancer, they should have told me.

Based on my most recent experiences at the HMO, I truly believe that they have written off dad. I wonder if they think that he has one foot in the grave so let us not waste time or our money since Medicare does not pay us enough. This is why I believe they keep pushing me to place him. I do not think they are doing it for me. I believe they are doing it for themselves.

I wrote both doctors (primary and geriatrics) and copied each of their supervisors. I want them to help as much as they can without the extra nonsense. I also wrote NCQA, CMRI, The Department of Managed Health Care, and my state politicians. Only time will tell what will happen. Right now, I am more than livid.

I also received a letter from legal, supposedly in response to my claim for the closet door my father fell into while on both Ativan and Haldol. She says the letter is in response to the one I wrote to membership services because I put a dollar amount in the letter. I really wonder if it is because I sent several letters to her boss.

My father's doctors received my letter and both their egos were bruised. The primary doctor said that he did tell me about the elevated white blood count, but only after I told him it was up to 40,000. Why did he not call me to let me know that the white count was l7.5 and why did he not follow it up with another blood test in about one or two months? The doctor stated (after I told him my father's white count was 40,000) that he thought the l7.5 was due to the Depakote. It was slightly higher than normal. He should have repeated the blood work a month or two later to confirm.

The doctor also said if I wanted him to know about the test results, I needed to call him. Since he does not get the results from the Valley facility, I had to tell him. Hello, I told him about the tests. DUH! I also told the doctors in ER to send copies to his primary doctor. Of course, they should have sent the results automatically. What? Fax machines do not talk to each other? If it was not so serious, I would laugh. Does the doctor have a telephone? Sure, he does. I do not see any reason why he did not call and get the results.

He agreed that someone should have followed up the chest x-ray. He is my father's primary doctor. He should have called to get the test results. There are times I really want to hit my head against the wall. This is so illogical.

I talked to member services again. I wrote it in letter form and sent copies to NCQA, CMRI, legal, my politicians, and the Department of Managed Health Care. Enough already!

All I can say, this is a hell of a way to run an HMO.

I sent an e-mail to member services. I received a phone call from someone who only identified herself as being from member services. She wanted to speak to my father to see if he wanted to continue the claim against his doctor.

I told her that my father had severe dementia, was disabled, and was taking a nap. She could not talk to him. I also told her that I had power of attorney.

She started to argue with me and insisted that she talk to my father. The more she insisted, the angrier I became. I did not scream at her, which surprised me, since I was so close to erupting. However, I held my ground.

I asked to speak to a supervisor. She told me there was no

supervisor on duty. I find that hard to believe. However, I asked to have the supervisor call me back.

Approximately fifteen minutes later, a supervisor called. I told her only a small portion of the problem that had increased my stress levels.

I also mentioned that I was tired of being a "walking file cabinet" and teaching people how to do their jobs. She actually finished my sentence after I said teaching. I know she "got it." Now, if the rest of the employees would "get it!"

She apologized and said she understood. She told me that she was going to talk to the employee and since my father was not going back to the doctor, she would send the information about the doctor to the Chief.

I told her that I was seriously considering taking him out of the HMO for good because of all of the nonsense I have had to put up with and should not have had to deal with at all. Frankly, I am tired of fighting against the lack of quality care, bad interpersonal skills, lack of compassion, etc., and having to continually fight against brick walls.

Today, when I arrived home from seeing the surgeon, an employee from the HMO called to follow up my complaint. She said she would send it to the Chief but only after she contacted legal and asked if she could file the complaint since I filed a claim with legal.

We talked about what happened regarding my father's primary doctor. I told her that the one facility never faxed the results to the primary physician and the primary doctor never called to obtain the test results. I told her it is a hell of a way to run an HMO.

She said she understood my frustration. She was not the only employee to tell me I had to do what is best for me, my father, and my sanity. I agreed.

I also took him into the surgeon for his three month follow up appointment. The surgeon said he was doing well, all things considered. I like him. He wants to see my father back in six months.

I told him my father may be out of Kaiser and I told him why. He sort of looked at me and shook his head. He also gave me the names of three doctors in the facility where we went and told me to contact them. I will contact the three doctors the surgeon recommended but at the same time, I am going to keep my options open regarding the use of Medicare and Medi-Cal.

In the meantime, I had a long talk with one of the nurses. She is a family caregiver for a parent with Alzheimer's disease. The parent is on Medicare and Medi-Cal and there are not any problems with care, just the social worker. Hopefully, I will be able to have a good social worker to deal with all of the issues because the HMO is not a lot of help. The nurse definitely heard my frustration and shook her head. I told her to read my website. She would find it interesting.

I do not know how much time my father has left, but I need it to be as stress free as possible for both of us.

As I might have mentioned, I wrote to the doctors on the surgeon's list and to the doctors whose profiles (dates of internships, residency, picture, school) the HMO sent to me for review. I did not find the profiles very helpful, as there was not enough information on which to base a solid decision.

Today, I found out one of the doctors sent my letter to the patient representative at the HMO. In the letter I stated that I wanted a doctor who was compassionate, caring, knowledgeable, pays attention to detail and follow through, and will fight the Utilization Review Board, if necessary.

The patient representative called. She told me that the "Utilization Review Board is made up of our doctors." What does that have to do with his primary doctor fighting the Utilization Review Board? It is almost as if she was saying that since the HMO's doctors make up the Utilization Review Board, there is no reason for any doctor to "fight them." To that I say, "Baloney."

If a doctor agrees that a 24 hour stay in the hospital after major dental surgery on an 87 year old man is reasonable and the Utilization Review Board says no way, the doctor should be able to say that he thinks it is necessary. To me, it sounds as if the HMO is trying to save money at the expense of the patient.

I briefly told the "patient representative" (in title only, of course) some of the things that have happened. Her reply, "If you have that many complaints, go to membership services or go to the Department Administrator," as if that is going to do any good. Been there, done that, and wore the T-shirt for almost four years. Has anything changed? I have not seen anything that remotely looks like real changes. I see only cosmetic ones.

I do not know what the HMO's definition of a patient representative is, but I know how I would define it. Her responses did not even come close, which is why I called her a patient representative only in title.

I really become so tired of having to teach HMO employees and others how to do their jobs. This is just another on the list.

I reported this patient representative several years ago for her attitude and lack of customer service orientation. I see I have to do it again. I wrote membership services and told them to contact the supervisor and have this person go to customer service training again. A patient representative who does not represent the patient! Par for the course.

Today, I received a phone call from someone in member services. In reality, she was from the department that takes the phone calls. Listed below is the way she began the phone call. Is it any wonder, I have to "train" their employees in the "art" of customer service so I do not have to "jump through hoops" to get the so-called quality service they frequently advertise.

She begins the conversation by saying, I am so and so (I do not remember if she mentioned the name of the HMO but I remember everything else). I received a message regarding a voice mail you left about (a person's name, which she got wrong). I asked her if she was from Administration. She said, no and that she was from member services. She did not give any more information than I just gave you. There are several member services departments. Then, I corrected the person's name and asked, how can the HMO keep a patient representative who is not properly doing her job? She replied, "That's not a complaint, that's a question." I said "No, and that is the complaint." She is not properly doing her job. This is the second time over the past number of years that I have had to complain about her. I added I am getting really tired of having to teach the (HMO) personnel how to do their jobs. That one went right over the employee's head. Figures.

I sent an e-mail to the supervisor of that department and said listed below is how the conversation should have gone and it would have if the employees were properly trained in the "art" of customer service.

"I am so and so from (name of the HMO) and I am calling you in response to a voice mail message you left on (name of the department's machine). The department employee forwarded the message to me. You have a complaint against (name of person). How may I help you today?"

In regard to the question/complaint, she should have said, "Let me repeat this back to you to make sure I understand it" or "I am going to repeat this back to you for clarification. Are you saying that the patient representative is not properly doing her job?" I would have said yes and the matter would have been a more pleasant experience.

A representative from membership services called. We spoke about the various and newest problems I was experiencing. I told her about the patient representative and the employee from the call center. She brought up a very interesting point-one that I had been too busy to think about. She told me that the employee in Administration could have called me to ask if I had resolved the issue or had contacted anybody else in the two days she was out of the office. I left the message on Tuesday and I e-mailed member services on Thursday.

She also told me that radiology does not send the results to the primary doctor unless it concerns a pediatric case. Everything is entered into the computer so the doctor can call up the results at any time. I asked her what happens when the primary doctor is not at this facility and not connected to this network system? She said she had to find out the answer.

I also told her my father's primary doctor did not bother to follow up the results of the tests since he cannot access the information in that facility's computers and that he had turned things around to say that I never told him. Is this great service? You could fool me.

I mentioned that I was sorry for "screaming" in my letter to her co-worker but I am so frustrated by the responses I receive that I really am getting tired of fighting this hospital. I told her that my father was incoherent and mumbling on Monday and Tuesday following the trip to ER on Sunday in which the doctor gave him the medication. He got up Tuesday long enough to holler in pain and when a regular hospital sent him home in an ambulance Tuesday night, and the employees placed my dad on his bed, he stayed there until Thursday afternoon. Dad woke up long enough to eat and drink and promptly went back to sleep.

I also mentioned that as soon as I get my father's Medi-Cal card straightened out, I was really thinking of taking him out of the HMO. It is too big and I doubt I will ever get the service that the HMO keeps advertising.

I received the customary letter from the member services representative. The letter stated that ER does not send the test results of test to doctors unless the patient is referred by a doctor. It is the HMO's policy. My father did not have a referring doctor at the time of the test. The paramedics suggested I bring him into the HMO. Therefore, the results should have been sent to the primary physician. This is just common sense.

The member services representative also stated that the doctor can check the computer to obtain results. I told her during our conversation that my father's primary doctor could not check the computer because he was not networked to that particular computer system. She never mentioned anything about that in the letter. How interesting!

I also thought it was quite interesting that disabled patients had to file a class action suit about the comments they received from doctors and nurses at one of the branches. This was written in one of our newpapers. The situation never should have gone that far.

I also mentioned that both situations made the HMO look stupid.

Today, the legal representative sent me a letter stating that they did not find liability in anything the HMO did or didn't do from 1997-Present. Please, give me a break! The HMO did not take responsibility for anything that it did or did not do. I knew they would not claim responsibility. I think the HMO has illogical priorities. The inane comments and lack of sensitivity among doctors, nurses, and social workers were bad enough. It is adding an insult to injury, that there were also problems with attention to detail and follow through, diagnosis, and everything else I mentioned in this chapter.

My father, under combined medication prescribed over the phone made him drowsier, so that he fell into the closet door, and the HMO is not responsible? The doctor, of course, did not write anything down in my father's chart. This is par for the course. It happened to me with my iron problem and now it is happening to my father.

My father, under the influence of 7.5mg of Haldol or more and 1 mg of Ativan injected directly into his bloodstream, sleeps on (mostly on) and off for 4 days, will not eat or drink (except for very little), has a seizure, loses weight, does not get enough nourishment or liquids because he cannot keep awake, is incoherent, mumbles, cannot walk without almost falling on his head, has all the classic signs of a drug overdose, declines in health, and the "thing" on his lung that nobody knew what it was two months ago, is now being called a nodule, and the HMO is not responsible? Oh, I almost forgot one. The case manager makes an inane comment criticizing me about my father's six pound weight loss but does not find the real reason (cancer) behind the weight loss and the HMO is not responsible? Excuse me, there is something wrong with this picture. But then, nothing about the HMO surprises me. The only reason my father is alive is because of my advocating skills, common sense, and persistence. If he did not have me to fight for him, he would probably be dead. He may not realize it, but he is lucky he has me to advocate on his behalf. The HMO made me angry one too many times. It is time for me to get my father out of it.

I do not know what I am going to do yet regarding action. I could go to arbitration. I would also like to file a class action suit on behalf of my father due to the inane comments many of the employees made. I would force the facilities' employees where my father had dental surgery, the clinic, and the one in the Valley to undergo sensitivity training.

I had to "train" another HMO employee today. God, I am getting so tired of the nonsense. If the HMO only listened! My father has an appointment at the HMO for the chest CT scan on May 21, 2001.

Our appointment to see the hematologist is May 22, 2001. We will go together. I set it up this way.

Driving to the HMO two days in a row is too much. The drive is approximately 13 miles one way. I called Specialty Services to try and change both appointments. The following ensued.

"Hello, my name is Eden and I would like to change my father's and my appointments from May 22, to May 21." The receptionist asked for my father's medical records number. I gave her dad's number and I started to give her mine. She sarcastically said, "Why do I need yours, this is just for your father isn't it?" I told her no. In fact, I explained that both of us had the appointment several times. Finally, I became frustrated and asked to leave a message for one of the nurses. I told her the message and she said, "Got it!"

She did not "get it!" at all. The nurse called back and said, "You want to change your father's appointment?" I told her I wanted to change both of our appointments to the 21st.

Nothing this HMO does or does not do surprises me any

more. The receptionist could not even take a simple message correctly.

This is scary and I shudder to think what might happen if the message was more complicated or a lot more important.

I sent an e-mail to member services at the call center. I wonder what kind of response I will get from member services.

I called the HMO regarding bad customer service again. I contacted the call center because the employees royally screwed up regarding my co-payments every month. They did not properly enter the information on this particular financial program. So they told me I needed to pay my $204.00 co-payment.

I immediately called member services on April 23, 2001. I spoke to a very nice representative who said she would take care of it. Apparently, the information had not been entered on one screen but was on another. Computer glitch or human error? It remains to be seen. However, it cost me time and effort to call again.

On May 1, 2001, I received another letter dated April 28, 2001. It stated my account had been terminated as of April 1. I did everything in my power not to erupt and I was pretty calm until I spoke to another employee about which I had to complain.

I told the employee that I wanted to speak to a supervisor. She asked me three times if she could help me. Each time I stated I wanted to speak to a supervisor. She asked for the details. I told her. She looked at my account and said it was fine. I asked her about the April 28, 2001 letter. She had not listened to one word I said. If she listened to me, she would have heard I spoke to a co-worker in the department who said she would take care of it. There was not one word mentioned that I had written. Earlier, I had already sized her up in regard to lack of customer service skills, which is why I asked for a supervisor. The employee transferred me and we became disconnected. I called back and got someone else. She transferred me too, but before she did, she took my phone number.

I complained about the employee and some of the things the HMO did to my father and me. I commended the one who took my phone number and did not leave me hanging. I also told her to get the appropriate people to fix their phones so when people do not get a person's phone number, the person does not have to call again.

I was not planning on doing a third book but with all of the nonsense happening, it just might be prudent. It depends on how fast my father declines.

An employee's bad interpersonal skills, lack of knowledge and follow through are a reflection on the HMO. I keep asking them why they do not "get it." It is so simple. Yes, I know I am dealing with human beings and human beings are not perfect. However, they advertise that they have such wonderful customer service and give quality care. Not in my opinion. I have taught classes on improvement of customer service productivity and have written articles on the subject. I know when I get good service and when I do not. I rarely see good customer service.

Now on to Chapter Four— In-Home Agencies: The Problems Continue

CHAPTER FOUR

IN-HOME AGENCIES:
THE PROBLEMS CONTINUE

OY VEY!, as they say in Yiddish. I wonder if the agency's employees will ever get their act together. I do not know how much more I can take. Although I need the respite, it is no wonder I hated to give up control of my father's care.

My father's caregiver could not come on her regular day. Instead of Tuesday, December 5, 2000, she agreed to come Monday, December 4, 2000. She agreed to come at 1:00p.m. so I could run errands on my list and accomplish my tasks.

At l:30p.m., I called the agency. We traded Tuesday for Monday. She is supposed to be here. Where is she? The employee told me she would call the aide at home.

Approximately at l:40p.m., the aide called me. She came down with the chills and did not feel well. I called the agency and spoke to the same employee. She said the aide called the agency and told an employee the same thing.

The employee and I had a very long talk. She asked me if I had any hair left on my head. I told her I did but only because it was so thick. I also told her I felt very frustrated. I told her that the aide did not call me on her previous day to tell me she missed two busses. I mentioned that the aide said if she called me or the agency, she would not have any change for the bus. I was about to suggest (I suggested this in my original book) that the agency accept collect calls. The employee said "We accept collect calls." I told her to remind the aide that you have the policy in place.

I also mentioned my conversation with one of the staff employees regarding fairness (see original). I told her it was not fair when employees told me it was okay for me to be late and then lecture me when I am. I went through the entire list of gripes concerning the lack of fairness and service. At least, she agreed.

During our conversation, she also said that she wished the aide would learn how to drive. I almost said, what good is it if the employees are not paid enough to purchase reliable cars. However, I did not. In my original book, I mentioned an employee said that the agency does not pay enough to ask them to buy reliable cars.

I told the employee that the aide is good when she gets here, but getting here is the problem. I need someone reliable. She said, "Maybe we should tell her the starting time is an hour earlier." We both laughed. I told the employee that if I did not laugh I would cry. She said she would try to find someone for Tuesday, December 5, 2000. I said I would like someone to show up on time and who has common sense. I need someone who can follow very simple oral and written instructions. Then, I told her about the aide who discussed the silverware in great detail so she would get it right. Yet, she still got it wrong.

Later, she called me to tell me she could not find anybody for Tuesday. I told her to find me someone for Wednesday. She told me she would. She validated my feelings of frustration. Validation is great. However, I am supposed to be getting respite, not grief.

I spoke with the person at the nonprofit agency funding my 25 hours a month. She told me that the contract is with this agency, not the one I suggested. I told her I was getting sick and tired at the lack of customer service, dependability, and reliability. It was making my job as a caregiver more difficult.

The employee at the agency found someone for Wednesday. She crossed her fingers and so did I. We would like to see this new aide receive a compliment for a job well done rather than numerous criticisms.

I told the employee I did not think I was being picky. I wanted the employee to correctly do his or her job. She agreed.

The agency sent another aide. The aide was better, but that is not saying much. The aide could not properly put the bedspread on the bed. She put the side at the top so it hung over on the floor. I may have to get a bedspread that says, "This side up." The aide followed most of the instructions. However, there are a few items I will have to discuss with her if she returns to watch my father.

I am not sure if I will have the aide return. I need to find out what happened to a cup I used at breakfast. I could not find it when I returned home. I looked in all the cabinets. It was not there. I looked everywhere.

I have one cup very similar to it but I know the difference between the two. Actually, there are three cups which are very similar and now I only have two left. I did not break it at breakfast.

The aide returned. I asked her if she remembered where she put the cup I used at breakfast and left in the sink to be washed. She told me there was only one cup. She used it and put it back in the cabinet.

There were two cups. I used mine and my father used the other cup. She showed me the cup she used. It was similar but not the same one. I guess I will never know what happened to one of my favorite cups.

I told her several times not to let my cabinets go so that they bang. Did she listen? No! I reminded her again. Did she listen? No! What part of such an easy request did she not understand, especially since there is no language barrier?

My frustration with the agency is growing. The agency informed me that someone else would be here on Monday. Well, guess what? The aide never called or showed.

She was to arrive at l0:00a.m. At l0:30a.m., I called the agency. An employee said she would try to reach the aide. At 11:10a.m., I called the agency again. The employee could not reach the aide.

The employee asked me if I wanted her to find someone. I told her no. It was already after 11:00a.m. and I had things to do and people to see. I told her to switch it to Wednesday. I further reiterated that I was in the throes of moving. I really did not need the extra stress and problems the agency was causing me. Although I am not paying for the service, I am frustrated by the lack of it.

The aide who never showed Monday arrived today on time. However, I am still going to have to train her. She turned off the surge protector for the microwave oven and left it plugged in the socket. I do not know why she turned off the protector.

On another matter, she could not properly make the bed. One side of the blanket was on the top. The other side hung on the floor. She did the same thing to my father's bed. We could have tripped on the blankets. As I said, I should get a blanket or bedspread that has an arrow that says, "This side up."

She also gave my father a shower. She turned off the hot and cold but not the middle. I turned on the water to take a shower that night. I almost froze.

Besides the above, she was supposed to come the next day at 12:00p.m. to 5:00p.m. She told me 1:00p.m. to 5:00p.m. I said no, it is 12:00p.m. She arrived at 12:00p.m. We lived in a security building. She had to call me so I could let her in. She called and I buzzed her in but nothing happened. Instead of calling me again, she just stood outside doing nothing. I had to go out and get her. I told her about the bedding, the shower, and the microwave surge protector.

Regarding the shower, she told me my father tried to get out of the tub. She felt afraid he would slip. She was in a hurry to shut off the water. Then, I am guessing she forgot.

I asked her about the microwave oven. She said she put it on for two minutes. At one and a half minutes she said it would not shut off so she turned it off at the surge protector.

Do I really have to bang my head against the wall with everything I am experiencing? Of course, it did not shut off at one and a half minutes. She set it for 2. The best option, which I explained to her, was to turn the knob backwards until the bell rang.

Since my microwave is 20 years old, it is now starting to fall apart. I did not want to move it and purchased a new one.

This should be interesting. If the aides cannot operate a very simple microwave oven, how are they going to be able to use the new one?

She told me she would be in on Monday at 10:00a.m. to 2:00p.m. Monday was the day I was moving. I told her she was supposed to be there at 8:30a.m. and work until 4:30p.m.

The Wednesday before I moved, the regular caregiver could not come. The hospital changed her hours to the day shift. The hospital called at 6:00a.m. The agency's employee called me at 8:35a.m. to tell me the aide was not coming. She offered to find someone else. The employee did not call me, so by 9:40a.m, I called the agency and cancelled. I switched the hours to after the move and stated "She better be here; I am moving." I also learned that the aide did not come on Monday because she thought the job was on Wednesday.

What is it with these aides? If I was paying for the service, I would have fired the agency a long time ago and retained another one.

The agency sent another aide. I really do not know why the agency hires some of these aides.

I can understand a person can become lost. I even got lost one or two times. The aide called me to say she was lost. I gave her directions. She did not even call me by my correct name. Upon her arrival, she buzzed the manager's intercom instead of mine. She had the apartment number and my correct last name.

She put her purse on my dining room chair which is very plushy. I asked her to move her purse and she asked me where to put it. My father was very grumpy, became more agitated, and started yelling at me. All I could think of to say to her was, "I do not know." Before I could collect my thoughts and say "Give me a minute," she became very unprofessional. She sarcastically said, "I cannot work like this. I am leaving." I told her she could not leave. In the meantime, her unprofessional behavior agitated my father even more. He started to yell. I called the agency and while the aide stood right there, I complained. The staff employee had a very bad attitude. She told me to go somewhere else so I could find someone more to my liking.

Finding someone more to my liking is not the issue. It is a question of the lack of professional behavior and common sense.

I told the staff employee that I was in the throes of moving and under a lot of stress and that I wished somebody understood. I think I made my point, at least for the moment. She never said another word. However, it amazes me that they could not figure this out on their own. They deal with family caregivers on a daily basis. The aide stayed. She could not properly make the bed. She placed the top of the sheet on the side. She did not do anything except make his bed (which I had to redo when I returned home), fix his lunch, and assist him in the bathroom. She helped me carry boxes, although I would have preferred that she clean his commode. She did not.

The agency's lack of customer service increased my stress levels and it was so unnecessary. I doubt the employees will "get it." The CEO of the agency never responded to my letter.

The aide who could not get the times or the days straight came on moving day. She cleaned the commode but I had to tell her to get my father out of my hair. He was in the way of the movers.

She wanted to put things away in the new kitchen. However, I never got a chance to line all the kitchen cabinets. It is a good thing she stopped when she did. I would have had to take everything out. As it is, I had to remove more than a dozen rolls of paper towels she placed in the bottom cabinet. As much as I use those, I would have had to bend over. Nothing doing. Anyway, it is my house. I want it the way I need it.

I asked her to help me find my surge protectors. I said they were in a box. There were only two regular boxes. She told me she could not find them. They were in a box underneath the second box.

She never gave her husband, who picks her up, my new address. I did not have a working phone. I could have stayed for a few minutes while she walked a short half of block to the corner to call her husband. Since she had no way to reach him, I had to go to pick him up while she stayed with my father.

The aides are driving me crazy. They must want me in the psychiatric ward. I keep praying to God to please deliver me from plain stupidity. However, the agency keeps sending more and more aides about whom I have to wonder. This is a reflection on the agency but they do not seem to "get it."

I used to be sent out on assignments. I always found my own directions or people gave them to me. I always wrote them down. If I did not understand the directions, I always asked the person to repeat them. If I became lost and had to call, I only called once. If I became lost after that, I stopped at a gas station. I never called an employer that many times. One aide called me three times for directions. I tried to accomplish certain tasks before she arrived. Her calls only kept interrupting my work.

I could see someone making a "Freudian slip" once and call a she a he. However, she referred to my father as a she more than six times.

I told her what glass and cup to give my father. She, for some reason I will never know, gave my father water in a wine glass. He broke it. I had to go out and replace it. Fortunately, it was not expensive. However, I am angered by the fact she did not listen to simple instructions. I doubt I am going to get anything out of the agency.

The agency sent a different aide. I got another headache. This is ridiculous. The aide used a good hand towel as a washcloth. I was still home when she washed my father. I do not know why she could not ask if I had any washcloths or what she could use to wipe off my father.

Before I left, I told her I needed the boxes thrown out and which trash bin to use. Upon my return, she told me the garbage bin was full so she could not throw them away. She kept them in the apartment. I would have put them in front of the container. I also told her I had to wash clothes. I do not know if she misunderstood or did not listen or what. She did not wash the laundry; she put the dirty clothes back in the cabinet with the clean ones. I had to wash them along with the clean clothes they touched. If that was not enough, I had everything organized. She did not even put the one shirt with the long sleeved shirts. She placed it between several pairs of pants.

She placed a cup of soda on my wood coffee table. I told her to please get a coaster. She complied. However, she never put it back. She left it on the table for me to put back. I added, "If you take something, like a coaster, please put it back. I am not your maid." The aides are here to assist me. It is not the other way around. It seems that all the aides created more work for me.

I had to retype my Do and Do Not list for professional caregivers. The placement of some items changed when I moved. I still cannot believe I had to type this list in the first place. At least, I was able to finish it before she returned on her next day.

I am not the kind of person to give up easily. Fed up, I placed another call to the president of the agency to follow up my letter. He apologized for not returning my call. He was working on several projects. He has more to complete. We spoke briefly. He told me he rarely receives complaints about the office handling my account. He said out of 12 offices, this one was the best. He further stated the aides pass the test and go out. The agency does not know what they do or do not do until they get called. I briefly told him what I experienced.

If the office handling my account is the best, I shudder to think about the others. I offered to work out a deal to do customer service training. At any rate, he told me to call him in March.

I really do not know how many more times I want to put up with unnecessary customer service problems.

This time, a caregiver was supposed to be at my apartment at 9:00a.m. At 9:20a.m., I called the agency. Apparently, the caregiver called them in the morning.

The staff employee thanked me for my understanding. I guess since I did not yell, I understood. I told the employee I felt angry that nobody called me. She said, "We just found out this morning. We were busy." She continued, "We found someone for you. She will be there from 10:00a.m. to 3:00p.m. I told her that it was already 10:15a.m. and the caregiver was not here. I wonder if she is lost.

I called the agency again at 10:30a.m. The staff employee said she would page her.

The aide arrived at 10:45a.m. The agency gave her the wrong directions. She got lost. I would have appreciated a phone call. At least, she gave me an extra 15 minutes for my trouble. I needed the extra time.

This particular aide tried to put several bulky blankets on my typewriter stand and over my VCR and my stereo. She almost knocked everything over. I showed her where to put them. She made the bed back into a couch and I left shortly thereafter.

Just before I left, I helped my father in the bathroom. I used the urinal bottle. It prevents it from going everywhere. I also told her to clean the bathroom floor after my father goes because he usually does not get it in the toilet.

My father was clean when I left at approximately 9:30a.m. I changed him before I left. I am going to have to talk to her to see if she even tried to change my father and the last time she did. I told her he had been constipated and that I gave him stool softeners so he would probably have to go again.

I arrived home at 1:30p.m. Upon my return, I found the blankets and pillows on my end tables. She rearranged the items on the table. Yet, there was a lot of space on the coffee table. I do not understand why she did not put the bulky blankets on a table that had more room. I also use the arm of the sofa and lay the blankets over it without any problems.

At approximately 2:30p.m., I took my father into the kitchen to give him something to eat. He said he needed to go to the bathroom. I took him. Boy, did I get a surprise. He was soaking wet and had been sitting on his movement. I cleaned him up. While he sat on the toilet, he went again. No wonder he felt so lousy. Besides that, I have concerns. I do not know when or if she tried to change him and how many times.

People with Alzheimer's disease and vascular dementia become incontinent. They forget how to go to the bathroom. Incontinence is one of life's hassles when taking care of a loved one with that disease.

It is no wonder why I keep asking God to deliver me from professional caregiver stupidity. How can these people pass the tests for a Certified Nursing Assistant and Home Health Aide and not have one ounce of common sense?

The agency called to inform me that my new regular caregiver was not coming. She had a restless night and would come the next day.

I am sorry she had a restless night. However, I am not going to give her a lot of sympathy. For me, there have been many a restless night due to caregiving duties or noisy neighbors. I still awoke and went to work and I do now.

The agency called me again to tell me they found someone to cover for the other one. There was one catch, I had to give up time. The caregiver had to be at her other job by 2:30p.m. This meant I had to return by 2:00p.m.

The caregiver arrived at 9:40a.m., not 9:30a.m., as the employee told me. I called the aide and said I would be late. I arrived home about 10 minutes late. The employee said it was okay. She called her next job and said she would be a little late.

As usual, I had more work to do when I arrived home. She did not wipe the bathroom floor after my father went to the bathroom. She also tossed trash in the bathroom basket and did not even bother to empty it. I had to toss the bag in the trash.

Professional caregivers are supposed to make my life easier, not to create more work for me.

My regular caregiver returned. She was due to arrive at 9:30a.m. She called me at 9:11a.m. to tell me she was on her way but wanted to stop and get something to eat. She told me she was supposed to get here at 9:30a.m. I asked her if she would arrive at that time if she got something to eat. She told me probably not. I told her to come over as soon as she could. She arrived about 10 minutes late. This is difficult for me because when I tell people I will arrive at a certain time, I expect to arrive at that time.

I am going to have to talk with her about using my good hand towels as a washcloth to bathe my father.

Ironically, a guest towel was in its holder on the bathroom counter. She took one out of the linen closet and used it as a washcloth. The guest towels look very expensive. Where is the common sense? How could anybody not know that it was a guest towel and not a washcloth?

I was home while she prepared the bathroom. She asked me what she could put on the floor for him on which to step. I told her either the pink or beige bathmat, which were hanging on the shower door. Yet, she did not ask me whether or not I had a washcloth or what she could use. They just do not "get it."

My regular caregiver could not come today. She called at 8:15a.m. Her child was sick and she needed to take care of him. She said she wanted to come Saturday. I told her I had a commitment for Monday. A little while later, an employee called me to tell me they were trying to get someone to replace her. Approximately a half-hour later, she called to tell me she found someone. She would arrive about 11:00a.m.

She arrived on time. I told her to read the Do's and Do Not list. I know she did not read it because she did not follow directions. She did not follow the directions the first time she came here. She is also the one who jammed the extension wand into the crevice tool of the vacuum cleaner.

She put my father's protective disposable underwear on backwards. No wonder he kept wetting himself. She also put the dirty laundry in the bathtub.

I placed a new roll of toilet paper on the roller in the morning. I arrived at about 5:00p.m. The toilet paper was almost gone.

I know I am not the only family caregiver experiencing problems with in-home agencies. However, it is still very frustrating and our legislators need to do something about it.

Today, I was silently reminded as to why I do not want someone to put away my dishes until I have had a chance to view them. I have had aides place dirty dishes, etc. in nice clean cabinets. The glass had residue which appeared to be small pieces of food by the top of the cup. I soaked and rinsed the glass in hot water so it would be clean.

I have over-the-door hooks on my bathroom door. She tried to close the door and broke the hooks. I think when the agency sends me the bill for extra time, I am going to subtract the money owed for the hook which she broke. I should not have to pay for it.

Just another day in the life of a busy caregiver who has issues with which to contend.

The next time she came to take care of my father, I had to remind her to wipe her feet on my mats. This is just common sense.

She did not give my father his medication or put fiber in his juice. I had to do it.

She washed him and used my towel as a washcloth in spite of the fact this is on my written list for professional caregivers. She said, "I did not know if the towel was yours or his. I know you said to use paper towels but I used the towel to wash him."

Let us see here. An aide does not know which towel is his so she uses any towel even though I said to use paper towels. I also showed her which towels were his to use to dry him after either a sponge bath or a shower.

The paper towels are only used for sponge baths and work great. I told her unless she gave him a bath to use paper towels. Obviously, she did not listen. However, I have since bought wash cloths.

Again, she put the blankets on the floor. I wish she would stop doing it. My father sometimes leans against the blankets while stretching out on the couch. Besides, the only time I put my blankets on the floor is when I change my bed. It is only for a few minutes.

I am tired and angry. Taking care of dad is difficult enough without the extra stress from the agency that does not have its act together. I just arrived home from my follow up visit for my bruises. I wanted to relax. I was in a great deal of pain. The last people I wanted to hear from were those at the agency. Unfortunately, they called and managed to push my buttons as usual. No caregiver or anyone should be subjected to what they are doing to me. In fact, if it continues, I will fire them. Then, the nonprofit agency can find me a better agency.

One staff employee called to inform me I had gone past my allotted hours. She also said that the employees at the agency became confused as to the number of respite hours the nonprofit agency had given me.

Next, I received a phone call from the office manager who should not be the office manager. She had a very condescending and patronizing attitude and said they were deleting seven hours from my current month.

If this was not enough, the aide left a message. The last line of her message said, "Call me on my cell phone and I will explain it to you."

I erupted as if I was a volcano. I really hate it when people treat me as if I am stupid, are condescending and patronizing, and blame me or try to penalize me for things that are not my fault.

If I became confused by the nonprofit organization's payment vouchers, I would have called the nonprofit agency for confirmation or verification. Did the staff or the office manager call? No! This was their first stupid mistake.

The manager made another error when she told me what time the aide arrived and left. She could not even get the time right. The employee may not have informed everyone else and the manager, without having all the facts, now has egg on her face.

The manager made the third and most damaging customer

service mistake when she stated I would be penalized seven hours. She obviously does not understand the "art" of customer service.

The agency made several major mistakes, informed me of their confusion regarding the hours, and then tried to penalize me for their stupid mistakes.

Is it any wonder why I erupted and why I frequently ask to be delivered from caregiver agency stupidity?

I called the office and left a very angry message to relay to the office manager. I made my next phone call to the CEO at the corporate office and left a message with the on-call employee. I told her to have him call me the first thing Monday morning. I then placed a call to the nonprofit agency paying for my so-called respite. I left the message stating what happened and that the agency, not my father, would be the death of me. I also asked the nonprofit agency staff to do something, including firing the agency. My next call was to the aide. I became angry at her last line and I told her how I felt. I apologized for yelling. She said I should not have to go through this and agreed the agency should eat the seven hours they had taken away from me.

Personally, the agency should "eat" more than the seven hours. Their lack of customer service and stupidity caused me a lot of grief.

Monday should be very interesting because I have had it and it is definitely not going to continue. I will not let it.

I placed another phone call to the CEO. I told him I was not going to eat the seven hours since it was not my mistake. I also complained about the manager's condescending and patronizing attitude. He called while I was out of the apartment. I called him back. He did not return my call because he was busy. I placed other calls to him.

The employee came here. She again placed the blankets on the floor to get them out of the way. She placed a wet washcloth over my father's dry towels. I do not know what happened to my towel, but I found another in its place and mine was in the hamper.

I learned that the employees receive instructions on how to make beds, do their jobs, etc. Are these people not listening to the trainer? It makes me wonder. What kind of training are they receiving?

The aide told me that I should not be going through the experiences I have had with the office. She also told me something I already suspected. I suspected the manager does not treat her employees very well. She confirmed my suspicions. No wonder the aides do not care, do not want to work, and have bad attitudes. This also explains why the employees have negative attitudes.

I finally spoke to the CEO. He apologized but negated the apology with excuses. One of the excuses he used was that the agency was a nonprofit organization. To that, I say so what! What does being a nonprofit organization have to do with employees doing their jobs, having good interpersonal skills, and owning up to a mistake? He said service can be really good but when it is bad it is bad. Really? This is why he needs customer service training for all personnel. He really believes, generally speaking, that there is nothing wrong with the agency's customer service.

There are times I really want to bang my head against the wall. I do not call the experiences I have had with this agency good customer service. It is not because I taught improvement of customer service productivity, it is because it is common sense.

I feel sorry for the other clients who are probably getting the same kind of negative customer service but are too ill or infirm to do anything about it.

I do not see how the agency can say I have a total of 18 available hours in February. Playing devil's advocate for a minute, I am supposed to get 24 hours from the nonprofit organization providing respite. I am supposed to get another 8 hours from Title 3B unless they did away with that in February and nobody at the agency bothered to tell me. Of course, I am not surprised. They really do not have their act together.

The nonprofit organization's director called the office manager who said they would serve me all the way through February.

That is not possible if they are only giving me 18 hours. That is okay. I will tell everyone I meet what this agency has done to me. This is what disgruntled customers do-they tell everyone who will listen about their bad customer service experiences.

The manager told the director that we needed a higher level of care than they could provide. The aides have clients in worse shape than my father. What higher level of care? As I told the CEO, I do not think I am asking too much to have people show up or call if they cannot come, properly wash dishes, do their jobs, and have good interpersonal skills. If the agency thinks that I am asking too much, then they should not be in business. I have a right to expect these things out of any employee who works for one of these agencies. Any caregiver should. Pure and simple!

This is not finished yet. I sent a letter to the CEO regarding our conversation. I am not going to allow him to tell me that his customer service is usually good. Not from what I have experienced. At the end of February, I will be done with these people who have no clue as to what constitutes good customer service.

However, this brings a new set of problems. What do I do with my father? I really do not want to do what the agency suggested, which is find my own person to hire.

The caregiver called yesterday. She asked me, "Do you know that the 20th will be my last day?" I told her yes. We also confirmed the hours for February. The 20th I thought would be 3 hours and the 13th she would come for 5 hours. However, I asked her to switch the last 3 hours to the 13th and 5 hours to the 20th since the 20th is my court date regarding my landlord issues. She said, "Huh?" I had to explain it again.

I asked the caregiver what happened to my towel. She used it to dry my father because she forgot that my father's towels were on the other side. Then, she arbitrarily picked another towel. She created more work for me. I had to wash two towels.

I also find it amazing that when I did not want her to come early, she did. Today, I needed her to arrive approximately 10 minutes earlier. Instead, she arrived a few minutes late. Ironically, she said yesterday, she would arrive at 8:40a.m. I told her that 8:50a.m. was okay. She said she would try. Interesting. She could come at 8:40a.m. but not at 8:50a.m. Very strange! I do not know if she works for a hospital during the nighttime hours but still 8:40a.m. is 10 minutes earlier than 8:50a.m.

I do not know if she did what she did because she felt tired. However, she put my father's pants on backwards. The pants had a label in the back and a tie-string in the front and she still put them on the wrong way.

The caregiver called today at 8:30a.m. She has a kidney infection and has to go to the doctor. She said she would make up the three hours at the end of the month. During our conversation, she asked if I had anything important to accomplish. I only had to go to make money and buy food. The weather did not help the situation. I do not want to take my father out when it is raining "cats and dogs."

I had to call work and tell them I was not coming. However, I did tell them I would make calls from home for which I probably would not get paid.

The aide and a staff employee called to say that the aide had to take it easy the rest of the week. I understand when someone is sick. However, I became angry. The aide never informed the agency she would not be coming on Saturday. The aide knew she would not be able to come a week to two weeks beforehand. She told me several times that she would inform the agency. Obviously, she did not and if she did, then another employee dropped the ball. Fortunately, the agency was able to staff it.

It is the aide's job to inform her employers or co-workers if she is not going to be at the client's site. It is not the responsibility of the client or the family caregiver.

On another day, a staff employee from the agency called to say the second person they were going to send had to cancel. The aide could not start her car. My reaction to that statement was, "Oh shit!" The employee was going to try to find someone else.

At 10:00 a.m., I called and told the employee who answered

the phone to cancel. They had not been able to find anyone. I mentioned that by the time they did find someone I would have to leave and come back because we had an appointment at the HMO. So, now I have to settle for afternoon hours on a day that I really do not want.

I have talked to the employees and the manager about the importance of aides having reliable transportation. Now once again, the agency inconvenienced me.

Everyone has colds or the flu. Whatever happened to employees working in that particular field getting flu shots? They could not staff five other jobs.

However, I do find it ironic that they are bending over backwards to please me. Even the manager is being nice. I would like to think it was because of what I said to the CEO. I flatly and honestly told him that it was just as easy writing articles with names.

The new aide came Saturday for five hours so I could teach my caregiving class. I do not know how much experience she had prior to joining the particular agency. I think she felt uncomfortable because she kept laughing at things my father did and said. She was another one who kept telling me she thought my father was so cute. After awhile I grew tired of hearing just how cute is my father. I told the aide she could "Daddy-sit" any time for free and take care of him when he yelled, became agitated, asked many repetitive questions, or wanted to go home, etc. Then, he is not so cute. She told me he already subjected her to dementia mode behaviors and he was not so cute.

As you have already read, I experienced a lot of problems with the agency over hours. I returned home almost ten minutes late. Instead of giving me the paperwork to sign (She did not know that I needed to sign it), she sat on my living room floor not doing anything for fifteen minutes. I allowed it her to do it for a reason. I wanted to see what she would do in those last few minutes. I finally asked, "Do you have any paperwork for me to sign?"

The aide said something interesting which I will use if the

agency charges me for the extra 1/2 hour. The aide said somebody at work told her if I needed more hours to stay because I had hours coming to me.

I wonder if she was talking about the four hours through Title 3B. I do not have any additional hours. However, my regular caregiver will make up my regular four hours on a Thursday.

How come nobody in the agency communicates? Is it any wonder why the agency keeps making mistakes?

On other matters, she could not get my father to eat. He wanted cereal. She gave it to him. He did not feel like eating chicken and a baked potato.

She also read my Do and Do Not List for Professional Caregivers. On it, I have related silverware information. It says "Please place wooden spoon up and all other silverware facing toward the sink."

I found a silver spoon facing up in the strainer. Okay, it is only a spoon. However, what if the directions were of greater importance than which way the silverware faced? She is just another aide who cannot follow simple written instructions. Like many caregivers, I find it difficult to get good help.

On the caregiver's last day, she hung up my father's wet washcloth on his dry towels.

I filed a complaint against the in-home agency with the BBB. I asked to be reimbursed for an aide's phone call, mileage to bring an aide's husband back here, for an aide's lunch, the over the door hook another aide broke, and the broken wine glass. I know they did not intend to pay it. They did. I have a suspicion they paid because of my complaint to the BBB.

I also called the Home Health Agency hotline and left a message. I will be filing a complaint with that particular agency as well. They have not as yet returned my call. I finally reached a "live" person who referred me to the Los Angeles number. I encountered the same problem. Nobody is returning phone calls.

Today, I tried again. I spoke to a "live" and very nice person. I learned that it is a violation if aides do not show up or call. I told her what the aides did and did not do. So, they will investigate that complaint and look for other violations when they go to visit the in-home agencies.

I received too much stress from agency personnel from September through February. I do not want any family caregiver to experience what I did.

The manager at the Valley office of the in-home agency told me that they would eat the extra 24 hours since it was their mistake. Today, April 24, 2001, they sent me a bill for the entire amount.

I called the agency's billing department and spoke to someone not versed in customer service. He wanted to know how I got the CEO's name (like it matters) and told me, "Well, you used the service, didn't you?" I said "That is not the point. The point is the agency was eating it since they screwed up, not me." He said, "Well, I guess she (manager) changed her mind."

I called the nonprofit organization helping with the grant and told them what happened. Then, I sent a consumer complaint to one of our consumer advocates. Then, I called the Health and Human Services agency and once again, I am going to "hit" the BBB regarding this nonsense.

This agency should not even be in business. I really feel sorry for the rest of the clients who use it.

Next month should be interesting due to the new caregivers and the new agencies.

I met the new person today. I hope she works out okay. She was referred by a family member of a person who works at the nursing home where I am marketing director. We went over the Do and Do Not list and the paperwork. She starts tomorrow.

The new person came today. So far, so good. She even killed two bees that came out of the stove vent and into the apartment. She had more courage than me. I hate those things.

The new person seems to be working out. I will have to talk with her about a few things such as: not throwing out the prune juice bottles as they are recyclable, not using my towels to put under the pads on the couch in case dad gets it wet, etc. People create more work for me by using towels as a buffer. I wash enough laundry. I am going to leave her a note tomorrow and tell her to wash his dirty laundry.

She called me at 7:30a.m. to tell me she was ill and not coming. Her next day is now Friday, which is okay. However, she told me that if she could come before Friday, she would call.

Well, Friday came and went. I wonder if the caregiver is ill. I left two messages on her voice mail. She never returned my call. Her husband never called. She never came. I had to take my dad with me.

I took him out to lunch but I would have at least appreciated if the caregiver called to say she still felt ill and could not come.

It is hard to get good help! Arrrgghhh! I thought when I "hired" my own aide, I would not have problems. She is a good worker but how can anybody so good, be so inconsiderate?

I never heard from her. Tuesday morning, she was supposed to be here. I called at 9:55a.m. and spoke to her husband. He said she was still sleeping. I said she was supposed to be here this morning. He tells me to hold on and returns to the phone. He says she is still sick. I said, "Okay I will not count on her tomorrow." He said, "She is sick; that is why she did not come." I emphatically stated I am a client, I have things to accomplish during respite time, and I would have appreciated a phone call from somebody telling me she is sick and that she cannot come.

I am wondering if she is going to be here on Tuesday, which is her next work day. I also wonder if she will call to tell me if she is still sick.

I called the aide at home on Monday to find out whether or not she would come tomorrow. I left a message stating that she needed to call me if she was coming or not on Tuesday, her scheduled day. So far, I have not heard one word. I do not know how to plan tomorrow and whether or not I have to drag my dad with me to the beauty shop to take care of my "mop."

I called the aide's house this morning and got her answering machine. I left a message stating that if she was not coming back I needed her to let me know so I could hire someone else. She called me once and said she was ill and I have not heard from her in two weeks. I could not go to my beauty shop appointment because I did not have anybody to watch dad and he did not want to go with me.

So far, the aide still has not gotten back to me so I am now looking for someone to replace her. Two weeks and not one phone call from anybody. I wonder what the reaction will be when I call to say that I have her check.

Is this so difficult? What is with these aides? I was ten times more reliable at 12 years old when I began to babysit than the people with whom I have had to deal. It is so frustrating.

Remember, you provide a service. You really need to have someone call and cancel for you if you cannot do it yourself. It is good business and good for business.

If you do not do what I suggest, you will get the reputation that you are unreliable. If you are an aide or employee in an agency, I would like to remind you that good service is rarely talked about but bad service spreads like a fire. By not calling the client or by continually showing up late, you have already started to dig your own career grave. Besides, if you do not call or show up, you could be in violation of the law. Then, you can kiss your career good-bye. All it takes is one phone call to say, for example, "I am ill. I will not be coming for a week" or "I am not coming back."

I still have not heard anything from my caregiver. I am angry. I even left a message on her answering machine that I had her money. She still has not called me.

I stopped in the facility in which she works. She was not there yet so I left a note for her to call me regarding the money. She has not called me. As soon as I give her the check and we are all through with each other, I may report her to Human Services' licensing and certification agency, as it is a violation to not call and not come.

If I do not hear from her on Monday, I might have to stop into the facility in which she works and find out more information. I know she lives in Eagle Rock. At least, I have the check.

On Monday, she called me. She apologized. She said she was in an accident and had been running back and forth to the hospital. The nursing home sent her the note I left for her. She said her husband was supposed to call but obviously he did not call. She or her husband will pick up her check. Her husband picked up the check and the paperwork for his wife that she needs to sign.

At any rate, I had to hire someone for Saturday for two reasons. One, I am supposed to be teaching a class on how to survive being a family caregiver. Two, one of my former neighbors invited me to brunch and I really need some time off. I have not had any respite since April 3, 2001. The agency I called charges $15.00 an hour. Of course, the employees never see that. I wonder just how much the employees see of that $15.00 an hour. I hope this one is good. I really hate training help.

I called the nonprofit group handling the grant. They called an agency and the employee called me. I told him some of the problems I encountered. They are going to try and get me someone for Saturday so it will not cost me anything. Otherwise, I will have to pay over $100.00 to get the respite I am supposed to get.

The employee at the new agency called me. After I specifically told him that I needed someone for Saturday, he called and said "I found someone for Thursday; will that help? I said "Sure, but I do not need anybody right this second for Thursday. My main need is for Saturday." If I do not teach class, I still have the brunch. There is an arts and crafts show in a nearby park. I do not have any money, but I like to go and see whatever people bring to the arts and crafts show.

Yeah! The employee called again and said he found someone for Saturday from 10:00a.m to 6:00p.m.. This is my first full day out since September when I went to the Los Angeles County Fair in September, 2000. He also said he found someone for Monday for 5 hours. Thank God.

The aide was okay. She could improve on some items. On the

Do and Do Not list, I stated that the chicken needs to be heated before it is cut. She cut the chicken before she heated it. It gets dry that way.

Dad would not allow her to clean him and he gave her a hard time when she tried to change him. She also told me that someday I may have to put my father in a facility. I may, but in the meantime it is none of her business. She was hired to make my life easier. She certainly was not hired to tell what I should do with my father, not in the here and now and not in the future.

I do not know if she is trying to prepare me for the harshness of the world or the disease or my situation, but I have been in a kind of "hell" since my father fell down in 1995 and then continued to become lost in his car and decline since his broken hip in July 1997.

The aide the service sent today-well that is a whole different story. First, she became upset with me because of my, "please remove your shoes" sign on the door. She said to me, "I cannot work without shoes." I said nobody else had the problem. Then, before I could stop her, she (and I do not have a clue as to what she was thinking) stuck her foot (thank goodness she was wearing socks) in my thongs and said, "Are these slippers for me?" I told her "No, they are mine."

The aide did not read the Do and Do Not List and did not listen to what I told her to do. I told her to cut up three prunes and put them in his cereal. I also told her to give him prune juice for breakfast. She wanted my help in changing him. I know my dad can be a handful sometimes, but she is supposed to know how to manage any difficult behaviors that might arise during toileting procedures.

I know she did not read the list. On it I state that I do not want professional caregivers to put their purses on my furniture. She did.

I called the agency that sent her, requested that they do not send her again, and explained my reasons. I said, "You just do not come into somebody's house and assume shoes left by the door are for you." I would like to know where they get these people. Is it arrogance? Lack of common sense? I wonder and keep praying to be delivered from professional caregiver stupidity.

I would like our legislators to raise standards, criteria, and training methods for professional caregivers. They need to do it and the time is now. I should not be going through all of the nonsense from the aides who do not have common sense in their little finger. I wonder if there is a test for common sense. Someone should develop one because it is needed. Legislators, are you listening?

Now onto Chapter Five—Landlords, Tenants, And The Neighbors

CHAPTER FIVE

LANDLORDS, TENANTS,
AND THE NEIGHBORS

As you may remember, I discussed various communication issues in my original book concerning my neighbors, landlords, and other tenants.

Due to the fact the aide did not show, I had to ask a neighbor for help. I needed someone to watch my father while I ran to the store. Fortunately, she allowed me the time to run the errand.

During my tenancy in this building, my father wandered out of the unit several times.

Unfortunately, one day, I had to run a quick errand to the grocery store. Upon my return, my father was nowhere to be found.

I asked the owner if he had seen my father. He said my father was with his manager. He thought the manager had taken my father to his apartment.

The manager was not around but I spoke to his wife. My father was not in their apartment.

I returned to the garage area to speak to the owner. The manager was also there so I asked him if he had seen my father. My father was walking around the garage looking for me or my car.

I called the police and since my father is cognitively impaired, an officer immediately responded to my cry for help. He came out to take a report and stay with me.

Approximately three hours after I returned from the store, there was a knock on my door. A woman brought my father home. He had wandered six blocks away from the building. Fortunately, the only thing that became scraped was his hand.

I find it amazing that my father complains about how much his leg hurts and that he cannot walk very well. However, when he is in a "wandering mode," these complaints just fly out the window.

At any rate, I did not expect management to "daddy-sit" but when management knows a tenant is cognitively impaired and wanders, I expect management to take the tenant back to his or her unit. I do not expect management to allow him to go out of the door.

Why do I expect it? Because it is part and parcel of providing quality service to a disabled tenant's family.

On a different matter, in the original book, I mentioned that the landlord told us to vacate the apartment. The lawyers worked out a deal giving me until December 31, 2000, to get the hell (at least that is how I feel) out of the complex.

From September to December 2000, I searched for the apartment or guest house best suited for us. The units were either too small, too expensive, or not in Burbank.

Then, one day, I thought I finally found one. The units were one level. I would not have anybody on top of me, just the sides. However, the owner, who acted within his right, gave it to his niece. The apartment was taken off the market.

Later that afternoon, I called on another ad and went to see the unit the next day. Due to time constraints, I decided to go for it. The pluses were it was the front unit, covered parking, no common side walls, and a laundry room on the premises. The minuses were one bathroom, one bedroom, near a carport, no gated parking, no central air, teenagers in the building who smoke in the courtyard, and a toddler who occasionally runs around the upstairs walkway. This is just what I did not want because it made me unhappy at the other place.

I did not learn about the teenagers and the child until I brought the first month's rent and security deposit. I became angry. The day I saw the apartment, the manager told me it was a quiet building. She also told me I could walk through the courtyard any time day or night and it would be "like this."

However, at this particular time and day, it was not "like this." I talked to the manager. I asked if she knew about the tenants who smoked. She said she did. I told her that I was allergic to smoke. She said there was nothing she could do and told me another tenant was also allergic to the smoke.

Then I mentioned the child running around the upstairs walkway. The manager told me that running around the walkway twice was acceptable and that I should not be able to hear it in my apartment. The children at the other complex were not supposed to do it but did it anyway. The manager told me to call her and continued by saying that if I had peace of mind, she would have peace of mind. The only way I would have peace of mind is for her to stop the child from running around and yelling and for my upstairs neighbors to be quiet. I did not know just how noisy the upstairs tenants were until I moved in.

How can someone say the building is quiet when a parent plays with his child so the child screams and then runs around? It does not matter if the child runs around once, twice, or even half-way. This negates the statement the building is always quiet.

She told me not to be stressed. I told her that I was already stressed. I am nervous about moving. I do want a repeat of the incidents I endured for the last three and a half years plus. As a caregiver, I am tired and stressed. I did not look forward to the extra expense and hassle of moving. One does not really know about a building until one moves into the complex. No tenant is going to tell you the truth for fear of being evicted. I crossed my fingers.

I went over to the new place. I paid the first month's rent and security deposit. The payment took a big chunk out of my savings account.

There were cigarette butts in the walkway, in the courtyard, and in the ash tray.

I could hear the children in the park but they were not as noisy as I thought they would be.

There are things in this apartment that still need to be fixed and should have been fixed before I moved in.

Moving is such a pain in the "you know what." I hate moving. Being a family caregiver makes moving much more difficult.

I moved things little by little. However, the big day was December 18, 2000. I was already exhausted. Having to move was so unnecessary. If my former landlords were proactive, customer service oriented, had good interpersonal skills, and understood the caregiving process, my father and I would not have had to move. But then, this is why I wrote a book about apartment management.

On the day I moved, several neighbors stopped by to say goodbye. One thought I would be there until Christmas. Two tenants asked me why I was moving. I said I did not have a choice in the matter. One helped me by taking the trash to the bin. Another said she was sorry she was losing a good neighbor. Two others wished me well and gave me hugs.

As for the building next door to my now former building, the tenants rudely awakened me at 2:40a.m. The tenants were having another one of their late night parties. They were having fun. They did not care who they disturbed. They laughed, sang, yelled, conversed, and talked on the phone, to name just a few of the things they did. At 3:07a.m., I called the police.

However, I still needed my sleep. After three and a half years of constant parties and loud conversations, I grew tired of their nonsense and inconsideration. I was moving in two days. I was not going to let them deprive me of my sleep as they had done during my tenancy.

We all need sleep. Sleep replenishes our mind, body, and spirit. Family caregivers who care for someone on a 24/7/365 basis, do not get enough sleep. Noisy and inconsiderate neighbors compound the problem. Maybe someday they will learn the hard way, what it means to be a caregiver for a loved one who is chronically ill. Then, maybe they will have to beg their neighbors for the peace and quiet to which they are legally entitled.

I do not want to call my former landlord any negative names, but one comes to mind right now. Today, three weeks after the move, I received the Security Deposit Refund form. Only, I am not getting a refund. He is charging me. I really hate unethical landlords. I am sure mine will deny ever telling me, "Do not worry about the condition of the apartment." However, he charged me $105.00 to clean the apartment. I was there over three and a half years. I did not leave the place filthy. In fact, the kitchen is cleaner than when I moved in. The kitchen was so full of cooking grease from Mexican food, I had to scrub and rescrub the vent over the stove. They sent out a "professional" person to clean it. Even after the person who came and cleaned it a second time, I found food items that could only be associated with Mexican cooking underneath the stove.

The landlord also charged me for replacing the carpeting. Any landlord who puts carpeting down in the dining area is asking for problems. The carpeting was over 3 years 7 months old. It was worn in spots and it buckled in the hallway, in the dining area, and the living room. My father could have tripped over the buckling carpet. Management needed to replace it anyway.

I find it ironic that when my father fell into the closet door they were going to replace the door while I was a tenant. However, now that I moved, I find it quite interesting that they are charging me. I plan to go into small claims court and file a lawsuit for the deposit as well as the severe water stains and mold in my father's closet.

As far as the mold goes, I wish I had seen the news segment on one of the local stations regarding mold and its dangers before I went into court. The news broadcast further stated that landlords need to take immediate action and care of the water problems before the water damage causes mold.

I would like you to think about something for a minute. What if your tenant was the one who wrote to the TV stations or called a press conference? What if the news reporter interviewed the tenant? You and your building would receive a very poor reputation. You do not want that to happen. That might have happened if the elderly tenant had become sicker than just having an allergic reaction to the mold.

At any rate, I sent a letter briefly explaining the mold and water damage, and that we had to endure it for three months.

I filed in small claims court and we went to court on February 20, 2001. I did not win, but I hope I showed him that I am a force with which to be reckoned. As I said, I really hate unethical landlords. Do not mess with me. I can become a real bitch when I have to fight against injustice.

Court was a story in itself and will be covered in another chapter in this book. My former landlord said a few things that were not true. He told the Commissioner that he had fixed the air conditioner system in July when, in reality, it leaked from July to September. The truth of the matter is that it started leaking in May. He stopped it and it started again in July.

My former landlord said he treated me fairly. I do not think he did. He evicted us because I exercised my rights. He told me not to worry about the condition of the apartment, the carpet, or the closet door. He could have done, what is called in Yiddish, a mitzvah, a good deed, and let us off the hook. After all, my father is sick, his former manager misrepresented the building, lied to the tenants, and admitted it to the owner when the owner confronted him. He should have let certain items slide.

The way I was treated depended on whether or not I was a favored tenant or persona non-grata, which is what I became after telling a relative of the manager's girlfriend not to run in the courtyard. As a favored tenant, he told me not to worry about the condition of the apartment. Once I became a persona non-grata, he charged me for the very items he told me not to worry about during various conversations.

My father suffers from sundowners (becomes more anxious,

agitated, and confused during the evening and nighttime hours). Noise bothers those with dementia. I had every right to tell people to please be quiet.

I also had every right to try and obtain a speaking engagement at any company I chose. I have a right to make money. I contacted the company for which the manager worked. As a speaker and author, I was worried that he treated his employees the same way he treated me. There are too many similarities between managing a department and managing an apartment. That day, I received my 30 day notice. Ironic, is it not? Reasonable doubt?

I really hope my books and the script sell. I have come to the point that the only landlord with which I want to deal is me.

I called the FHA of Housing and Urban Development. I wanted to see what landlords needed to do. I spoke about the grab bars and the landlord not wanting to put them in. He made comments such as, if the (name of nonprofit agency) wants to help you let them get you someone. There is no guarantee that your father would grab the bars. I do not know who would be doing the installation. The tub is made of porcelain. I would not want you to incur expenses taking it out. The landlord would not let me take off the shower door and put up a curtain because he would have had to throw out the doors.

There are two guarantees in life. Those are death and taxes. The nonprofit agency would have handled the installation of the grab bars, if the owner allowed it. The agency would have given him a copy of the contractor's license. The nonprofit organization does this all the time for others. Since it is already in, you could leave the grab bars there for the next person. I have been dizzy in the shower; I would have liked grab bars for myself. As for the door, it fell off the track and they put it back on the track without any problems. However, the owner said if they took off the doors, he would have to throw them in the garbage. They could have stored the doors downstairs in the parking area. They would not have had to take off the track.

Landlords make my job as a family caregiver more difficult.

When landlords tell me a building is quiet, I expect it to be quiet. New Webster's Pocket Dictionary defines quiet as "at rest" and "silence." Therefore, a building in which a toddler runs around the upstairs walkway or that has tenants playing their TV, etc. at 1:00a.m. loud enough for me to hear is not a quiet building. It is contradictory to the standard definition.

I never would have rented an apartment in a building where a tenant's granddaughter and a toddler were running around the upstairs walkway. If I had seen that and the manager told me it was a quiet building, I would have run the other way and hoped I would have found something before December 31, 2000.

To add insult to injury, I still do not have hot water pressure in the bathroom sink, a window that locks, and a new front door. The second smoke detector has not yet been fixed. This could be in violation of the law.

I hope I get the new door and window soon. They really need to do something about the flopping floorboards and the lack of hot water pressure in the bathroom. I hope I do not have to get tough.

I already hate apartment living. I am beginning to hate my new apartment. One of the neighbors turned up the bass. I hate the sound of a low level bass on a stereo. It is so annoying.

Another tenant left her clothes in the washer for a very long time. I had to take out her clothes. At least when I took them out, I shook them and laid them neatly on the table. I was a few minutes late because I had to help my father with his bathroom needs. A tenant took out my clothes and just tossed them any which way on the table.

I sent a letter to the manager because I am quickly tiring of these unnecessary problems. I am sure I will find the reply interesting.

The manager called me today regarding my letter. She said I would be getting the door soon but she was not sure of when the painter could paint it. I told her at least the door would be free of splinters. She also said he would bring the new window soon. As for the screen in the bedroom, she would have him nail it to the window.

The manager is also allowing the children to run on the upstairs walkways. This creates noise and is a safety hazard. It means it is really not a quiet building. She admitted her granddaughters were on the walkway, although she told me the youngest could not be downstairs in the courtyard because she would run away. She did not know who ran around the upstairs walkway at 8:45a.m. I told her I thought it was the toddler in the building.

Regarding the stereo, TV, etc., she said she would talk to them. She told me they were young, did not have any parties, and were being reasonable.

Sorry, but being reasonable is not just about having parties somewhere else. They do not have parties because management does not allow parties on the premises. Being reasonable is about consideration and not playing your equipment loud enough to be heard in somebody else's bedroom at 1:00a.m.

I spoke to one of the upstairs neighbors. She told me that they have parties every three to six months. So, they do not have parties? Parties every three to six months are a lot of parties especially when considering that the manager supposedly does not allow parties in the building and that the manager told me they do not have parties. Please!

One of the tenants approached me to tell me they were going to have people over the end of the week. In other words, they were going to have a party.

I expected noise (toilets flushing, showers, low level conversations) but not stereos, televisions, and video games at 1:00a.m. or children running around the upstairs walkway. I guess I moved into the wrong building.

The manager asked me how I was feeling. I told her what my father did to me when I tried to stop him from going out the front door. She said she tried to reach me to see how I felt. I told her I was on the Internet. I would sure like her to do something with my upstairs neighbors.

Last night, the upstairs neighbors were hammering from 11:20p.m. to 11:30p.m.

Tonight, they had their bass on the stereo tuned up quite loudly; my father even heard it. One of these days, I am going to call the police. They were spoken to twice and they still do not get it. Obviously, they only care about themselves.

I had to call the manager again. From 8:30p.m.to 8:45p.m., my upstairs neighbors were playing their stereo quite loudly. I could hear it all through the apartment. The driving drumbeat and bass gave me a headache. My father is hard of hearing and it bothered him.

I asked the manager if I needed to call the police because the stereo was so loud and that I heard the radio at 11:45p.m. the night before. The manager told me she spoke to them and told them to quiet down and not play anything after 11:00p.m.

The manager told me she talked to the upstairs tenants who apologized for the loud videos. Their excuse was that they had guests and they were showing off the new videos. The manager also told me that if they got too loud, I could come up and knock on the tenant's door.

Yeah right! I am not going to walk outside in my pajamas at 12:l5a.m. when they play their TV or stereo loud enough to be heard in my apartment. I will not walk outside to go to their apartment when it is raining. I did too much of that when I lived in my former apartment.

I find it difficult to accept their apology. They were trying to impress their friends. I am too tired and too stressed to fool around with people who do not understand how to live in an apartment complex. They have fun at the expense of the other tenant's quiet enjoyment of the premises. I knew college students who were a lot more mature and considerate and would not do some of the things these tenants have done.

At 3:00a.m., I heard music coming from the area over my bathroom. The upstairs tenants were playing the radio. At least, I only heard it in my bathroom and not in my bedroom.

Well, my upstairs neighbors did not heed the rules. I heard their TV or radio in my bedroom until 12:15 a.m. The manager told me they were not supposed to play any sound equipment after 11:00p.m. So, why did I hear their TV and or radio until 12:15a.m.? That is 1 hour and 15 minutes past the 11:00p.m. deadline. Although the music was only loud enough to be annoying, I would have preferred not to listen to it at all, especially when I was trying to sleep.

Again, I will have to speak to the manager.

I am not surprised that my upstairs neighbors used their treadmill at 3:00a.m. when they came home. It is so inconsiderate.

Later that night, someone parked in the driveway at 11:00p.m., blasting the bass on their car stereo. Again, how inconsiderate.

I am frustrated by the entire situation. Maybe I should write a "How To" (how to be a good and considerate tenant) book for tenants. I wonder if they would even "get it." Probably not! In order to "get it," they would have to care about someone else. They do not.

It is for the above and for other reasons why I wrote the original, this sequel, as well as "How To Improve Customer Service and Increase Profits: A Common Sense Approach To Apartment Management And Ownership." Apartment managers and owners really need help. I am too tired and too stressed to deal with any more problems from apartment managers and inconsiderate tenants. Enough is enough!

I finally got my new kitchen window. Too bad the worker could not install it when it was warmer. It got cold in here. He left a mess on the window sill. He had to come back the next day to caulk the sill and the window.

I cannot be too upset at him. He is going to return as a favor to me and put my closet door on its track. So he said. He never returned. He also put the blinds back crooked. Finally, the manager was here on Friday, having it fixed.

I ran into her a few days later and she asked me if there was anything else. Just the closet door, the bedroom screen, the hot water in the bathroom, the floorboards, which are getting worse all the time, and of course, a front door.

Also, my upstairs neighbors were "at it" again, playing their loud video games, etc. until 11:30 at night. It is 11:45p.m. and they are talking very loudly. I would like to see someone much quieter upstairs. I need quiet. I guess I will mention this to the manager and see if she will do anything with them. Otherwise, I am going to call the police.

I wish they would just grow up and stop making life miserable for me and my father. Dementia patients become agitated at loud noises. They have already disturbed dad by walking so heavily on their floor. I know they can walk lightly. They have done it several times. They should be able to do it all the time. If they do not start flying right, then I will call the Burbank Police.

I called the manager's son to ask if he could "daddy-sit" for me while I ran errands. One son was not at home and the other could not do it. He sent over two teenagers. One used to sit with a woman who had Alzheimer's disease. I had only planned to be gone an hour but since I had not run errands for over a week, I took longer. However, before I left, I told them I had a lot of errands to run and if I returned late, I would pay them a little more money.

At my last stop, I called home. The manager's son answered the phone and said the kids left, that his mother sat here for awhile, and he did too. However, he was not real happy that he and his mother had missed their appointments. I told him that I told the kids that I would pay them more if I was late returning because I had a lot of errands to run. I further stated that they never mentioned that they had other things to do at a certain time.

Even as a baby-sitter at 12 years old (these teenagers are about 14-l6 years old), if someone said, "If I might be late, . . ." I would have replied, "I have to leave at such and such a time." At least, they were smart enough to get someone here to cover for them and did not leave my father home alone.

As if I do not have enough stress in my life, (ha ha), a bee, wasp, or hornet managed to get into the apartment. It was buzzing and flying all over the kitchen window. I could also hear the critters buzz in the vent over the stove. The critters must have gotten in that way or through a crack somewhere else. It finally stopped buzzing as it got dark outside.

I called the manager. She said she would take a look outside tomorrow and there are a lot of the critters because of all the foliage. She said she wouldn't call a bee exterminator for one bee (actually I think there is more than one) because the owner would be very angry with her. However, I would have liked someone to come over and remove the critter from my kitchen window. I really do not want the critter in here and if it stung either my dad or myself, the results could be disastrous.

Well, there were more bees in the apartment. The professional caregiver killed two of them.

I called the manager, who sent one of her sons to check out the bee situation. He opened the vent and one climbed out. He killed it. Several others were still in the vent, but at least they were dead.

Now there were enough bees in the pipe and in the apartment to warrant calling a "bee expert." I am glad that nobody got stung in the process.

The manager's son stopped by to say that the bee expert would be here in about an hour. He was here in less than an hour. He placed a piece of mesh over the vent and sprayed. He said I could still have one or two bees come out but if I had anymore to call him. He guaranteed the work for six months. He gave me his card.

The owner has seven buildings and he might have become upset at calling a bee expert for "one" bee. It cost about $100.00 for this guy to come out and take care of the problem. It has been my experience that there is usually more than one bee.

Well, another bee decided to find its way into my apartment. It was buzzing up a storm in the bathroom window. I took some ant and roach killer spray and zapped it. The result was one very dead bee. The bee expert told me I would have one or two bees in the apartment. If I saw more, I could give him a call as it was covered by the contract. One more and he will get a call. I cannot take the risk of getting stung and neither can dad.

Compare the above experience with one approximately twenty years ago. I lived in Panorama City. I had a bee problem. I only had one bee in the apartment and several were stuck in the stove pipe. I could hear them. The manager did not have any qualms about calling a bee person. He found a hive on the property on the other side of the building and had it removed. He did not call the owner to get it approved; he just took immediate action. In fact, he came over immediately to kill the bee that was buzzing around in my window.

If the manager had not called the bee person for only one bee, he would not have found the hive and everybody would have had a bee problem.

While living in another building, I had two mud wasps stuck between my screen and the window in my living room. I went outside and sprayed through the window. They died. Management called the exterminator. He found the nest buried in the dirt in the flower bed near the apartment.

Recently, I walked through the courtyard of the building in which I live. Someone was blasting their stereo or TV. I could not tell from which apartment the noise came. However, it sounded as if it came from the apartment next door from the manager.

The manager told me that "My courtyard is the quietest around. I do not let the music get louder than this (this was in reference to her own stereo)." This stereo was a lot louder than hers. I could not hear her stereo outside the apartment.

People need to be considerate. My upstairs neighbors were awake at 8:l5a.m. and playing music. It was not loud but I could still hear it in my bedroom.

The neighbors in the building next door were outside talking very loudly at 9:15a.m. Needless to say, I felt tired. Besides, I guess they do not care who overhears their conversations. It may be 9:15a.m., but there is absolutely no reason for them to be talking as loudly as they did. You have to be considerate of other people. Well, they look young. What can I say?

I am so glad I do not live off the courtyard. A few days ago, a small school bus that a small child can ride was left in the walkway coming into the courtyard. Today, two children, who appeared to be guests, were playing in the courtyard. One was over to side spooning something. The other was right in the middle of the courtyard playing with these little bikes. The courtyard is not too big. I just hope that if my father does wander out the door that these kids are not in the courtyard blocking walkways and paths. They are not supposed to be playing in the courtyard fixing bikes and tricycles, etc. It is a safety issue.

Today, the manager's granddaughter was outside on the walkway. The toddler started to make noise. I could not believe my ears when the manager and her son both yelled at the toddler one right after each other to stop the behavior. Then the child ran around the upstairs walkway.

The next day, a tenant's toddler and another small child, possibly the manager's granddaughter, were outside running around the courtyard screaming. One was running after the other one who was riding the tricycle. This is a safety hazard but I guess someone will have to get hurt before it changes. I just hope it isn't my dad.

I let the manager know that this disturbed me just after I moved into this apartment. By allowing her grandchild to run around the upstairs walkway even though it disturbs me and sometimes my father, she is putting out the non-verbal message, "I care more about my granddaughter's fun than about you being disturbed." As I previously mentioned, she believes that twice around the upstairs walkway and x number of minutes running around and yelling in the courtyard are okay. I do not.

Today, I met my former neighbor for lunch. She bought. I am very glad. It was also good to get outside. I walked to lunch. It is a three mile trip there and three miles back. I am surprised that my legs are not giving way. Anyway, lunch helped.

Caregivers need understanding neighbors, tenants, and land-lords to help them through a very difficult time.

Now onto Chapter Six—The Move

CHAPTER SIX

THE MOVE

I took my father to the new apartment several times. He did not want to see it. However, my father said he would be happy as long as he was with me. There might be a point where I will have to make a decision but for now he will be with me.

I know this move was hard on my father. I had to orient him to the new place. I found it to be a major effort, especially for the first two weeks, at the very least.

The move was difficult for me as well. Moving is extra work, expense, and hassle. Besides, the new apartment is only a one bedroom.

Do I have any regrets at what happened? Yes and no. I do not have any regrets leaving the hassles and the lack of customer service and ethics I had to endure, as well as getting away from the building next door with their continuous late night parties. I do not regret getting the "Hell out of Dodge."

I regret leaving the tenants with whom I built a rapport and became friends. I would like to visit but I am not sure I want to set foot on the property ever again. It has too many bad memories. Maybe someday, I will be able to forgive the management and owner for the hell they put me through knowing I am a family caregiver. However, right now I cannot. I am too angry and it hurts too much.

I walked through the old apartment with my former manager. He said is (owner's name) aware that the closet doors have been removed? I said yes, (owner) and (previous manager) took them off.

I wanted to see how they would handle the closet. Now, as I previously stated, they decided to charge me. How interesting since they were going to replace it with a mirrored door while I was a tenant. I told them for the sake of my father's safety and well being not to replace it in case he fell into it again. I did not want him to fall into the mirror.

Moving into the new place became more difficult than I thought and very scary to say the least. The knob on the oven was broken. The gas company turned on the gas in the new place. However, the oven became very hot. Due to the fire hazard, they turned off the gas. Supposedly, they only turned off the oven, not the gas for the whole apartment. However, I could not get the gas to work. Finally, I did and management gave me a brand new oven.

Besides the above, the fixtures had no light bulbs in them. I did not get a lot accomplished. I would have had to stand on a ladder to put the bulbs in the fixtures, but I did not. I felt afraid I would fall (I get dizzy at times) so I asked the manager. Eventually, they put the bulbs in the fixtures.

On another matter, I left two plungers at the old apartment in my haste to leave the "war zone." The plumbing in the old apartment was horrible. The toilet off the hallway always became stuffed no matter how little toilet paper we used. One day, management pulled out a big gob of long hair. Even so, it still got stuffed quite easily. So did the bathroom in the master bedroom but not as badly. The sinks became easily plugged. I forgot the plungers, but I hoped the new place did not have these problems.

It took me awhile to get the apartment in shape. Dad kept becoming more confused. He initiated the carpet. I am not surprised by my father's confusion and disorientation. I expected him to be confused. He found the move quite difficult and he still has not adjusted to the new place.

Tonight, December 30, 2000, was the first night my upstairs neighbors did not pump up the volume on their stereo, TV, and video games. They usually become too noisy. I asked the manager to tell them to keep it down, especially after 10:00p.m. I know why they were quiet. They were not home. They arrived at 2:00a.m. By 2:10a.m. they had already turned on their stereo or TV set.

The screens and windows need to be replaced or fixed. The apartment needs a new door which they were supposed to give me before I moved in the complex. I hope they fix the door very soon. There are splinters.

One Saturday night, I had to ask the manager's son to turn off the sprinklers. They were on at 5:00p.m. We could not get into the apartment.

It is now January 2001. We are finally settled in the new apartment. The only thing I have to accomplish is hanging my lamp. I asked a male friend if he would come over and help. He said he would.

I would be happier if my upstairs neighbors were considerate and turned down the volume on their TV, stereo, and video games without my having to complain. However, after what I experienced at the old place, I really do not want to put up with anybody's nonsense any more. Enough is enough!

It is now almost two months since we moved. My father is still not adjusting to the move. He keeps asking, "Where is my bed? Where do I sleep?" This is why you do not take a cognitively impaired person and move him or her as if he or she were a piece of furniture. It is very traumatic and unsettling to move elderly people and more so those with cognitive impairments.

Just after I moved in, I asked the manager to trim the bushes blocking the walkway. The manager said that there would be too many brown branches and they could not be cut. My father could have fallen down and broken an arm, hit his head, or broken the other hip. Needless to say, I would have became a raving lunatic and held management responsible.

One day I came home and found that the bushes had been cut back to their branches, and the sprinkler hole where my father usually almost trips was filled in with dirt. Will wonders never cease?

There were more wonders to come. There was one skinny tree left standing and the two bushes on each side were down to stumps.

I wish landlords would listen to their tenants. Tragedies, such as the one that happened to the manager who fell, could be prevented. How? By listening to a tenant who had a great idea.

Now the manager plans to cut down the foliage on the other side and replace it with slower growing plants and shrubs. This has already begun. I am glad that the bushes will be smaller. While it may have been slightly cooler with all the shrubbery, I felt worried that someone might someday hide in back of the bushes.

When my father fell, he hit his head on the stump. I wonder if it would have been easier or better if he hit dirt.

Three weeks after the fall, I returned home and noticed the bush stumps were gone. The gardener removed them. I wish they had been removed last month. If the stumps had been removed, my father would have hit soft dirt. I do not know if that is good or bad, but I do know he would not have hit the stump. He came so close to the stump that the branches were very near his eye and his ear. He was hurt enough, but he could have gotten severely injured due to the stump.

It should not have mattered if I was a new or an established tenant. What mattered was the growth of the plants and how they jutted out onto the walkway and the sprinkler holes. Both of these items should have been taken care of long before the manager fell.

Now onto Chapter Seven—Dealing With Court

CHAPTER SEVEN

DEALING WITH COURT

I cannot stand going to court but it is something I felt and believed I had to do. I filed against my former landlord and lost. I am angry. I am not angry because I lost. I feel angry at the way the Commissioner conducted business. I had a professional caregiver with me in court so she could handle my father. She even said, "I do not like the way he conducts business."

Since my days in court, I decided I was going to try to get the Commissioner recalled, taken off the bench, etc. so that no caregiver experiences what I did twice. I do not care how many landlord/tenant disputes he has handled, he is not good on the bench. Respect is earned; it is not a right or a privilege.

I maintained that the extensive water damage would have ruined the closet door if it had been installed. He knocked that down on the basis of it being an assumption. I also maintained that the mold put my father at risk and furthered his allergies. The literature from the California Health Department, Centers For Disease Control, etc. states that the elderly are at risk. This, coupled with the letter from my father's doctor, should have been enough. Not for the Commissioner. He said something about not knowing my father's medical condition so he could not use that information. Yet, he made plenty of assumptions when it suited him.

The owner stated that I ruined the rug (we're talking the complete rug) because my father was incontinent. My father has dementia, which the Commissioner said he understood. However, his next statement was the biggest assumption of all. He said, "I know about dementia so I am going to say that your father went all over the apartment."

I did everything (chewed on the stick of my pen) to control my temper in the courtroom. I became furious. I became livid. A volcano waiting to erupt might be better a description. I have lived with dementia for over three and a half years on a 24/7/365 basis. I do not know the Commissioner's experience, if any, with dementia but I will wager I know more about dementia than he does. I have done research and read a number of books.

If he knew anything about dementia, my father, or anything about my caregiving abilities, the Commissioner would have known that my father runs from alert to confused, that my father wears incontinence supplies, and all dementia patients are not the same nor do they exhibit the same behaviors. Dementia patients are unique unto themselves.

The Commissioner also made the statement that he did not know my father's medical condition which is why he could not rule regarding the allergies. Yet, he still made the remark that my father has gone all over the apartment. If he does not know my father's medical condition or history, then logically speaking, he could not make such a blatant generalization.

However, the clincher is that just a few months prior to this case, I was in his courtroom having him hear a case against an adult day care center. If he knew anything about dementia, he would not have made many of the statements he did.

I maintained the aides teasing my father, their defensive attitudes, and just as important, their lack of training, caused my father's catastrophic reactions. Their own log, which the adult day care personnel submitted to the Commissioner, proved my point. The log actually spoke volumes. This issue is primarily addressed in my original book.

The Commissioner did not understand that my father's combativeness was a reaction to the aides' attitudes and lack of training. I understood before I read the log because I witnessed some of the incidents. The log gave me insight and more proof. I have seen it with my own father in my treatment of him as to how responsive or combative is his behavior.

If the Commissioner really knew about dementia, he would not have said, "Your father has a problem." He also would not have said, "Maybe the aides need some training." Some? Please!

No, my father does not have a problem. He is a little, tired, elderly man with a horrible disease that continues to rob him of his memories, cognitive abilities, and his happiness. The day care center is the one with the problem for not knowing how to manage difficult behaviors that may or may not have appeared or my father in general, which I believed caused many of my father's difficult behaviors.

In both appearances, the Commissioner insulted my intelligence. Most recently, he told me the landlord was a businessman. Really, Duh!

I had my own business for five years in employer/employee relations, ethics, and improvement of customer service productivity. I spoke to many business people. Business people, if they are decent and ethical, have hearts, even small ones.

Also, I lived in an apartment for five years in North Hollywood. Approximately one year after I moved into the complex, I fell down and broke my ankle. I was in a cast for 10 weeks. After the doctor removed it, I headed for the shower. I was wobbly getting in and out of the tub. I fell against the glass door and cracked it. Did the owners charge me for the door? Not on your life. They did not charge me even when I left the premises for greener pastures and a one bedroom apartment. I am sure they wanted to make a profit like any other person who owns rental property.

The Commissioner also insulted my intelligence by giving me $10.00 a month for three months for "looking at the mold and the water stains."

Anybody with any common sense knows that you just do not look at mold for almost three months. It smells. I should not have had to say, "And gee your honor, it smells bad too." Give me a break!

The Commissioner also spent over five minutes talking about the stipulated agreement between me and my former landlord. I did not get a 30-day notice because of non payment of rent or for using the repair and deduct remedy (which I did not use). I received the 30-day notice because I exercised my rights.

Then, when I brought up a point, the Commissioner said, "We spent an hour on this case." Yet, when I was in court regarding the day care issue, he allowed a case to continue for 1 and a ½ hours. He said it was complicated. I did not find it that complicated and neither did the others who waited for their cases to be heard.

I think I made my points as to why the Commissioner should be removed from presiding over small claims court. Remember, respect is earned. It is not a right or a privilege. Nobody, especially a stressed out family caregiver, should be treated in the manner I was by anybody, including those dressed in black robes.

I wrote to his boss. I received a letter from the presiding judge. He agreed with the Commissioner. Why am I not surprised? The presiding judge ignored my argument that the Commissioner based his decision on one of his biggest assumptions which was that since my dad had dementia, he went everywhere. The Commissioner failed the "I know about dementia" test. The presiding judge also made the assumption that I wrote him to appeal the decision. Nowhere in my letter did I make that request. I wrote to him to complain. The presiding judge sent me the address for the Judicial Review Board in San Francisco. I sent them copies of the letters and the presiding judge's reply along with a letter disagreeing with the presiding judge's response. It will be interesting to hear their response. I wager they will side with the presiding judge. Gee whiz. Give me a break.

So far, I have not received a response from the Judicial Review Board. Maybe I will have to address it in the third book.

Now onto Chapter Eight—Dealing With The Government

CHAPTER EIGHT

DEALING WITH THE GOVERNMENT

I cannot believe the post office. I take that back. Yes, I can.

I ordered a coffee mug of one my pictures that won a semi-finalist award. The mug came. I have not been able to see it yet.

The mailman put it in the mailbox. Since the boxes are larger at the top, he slipped the box in to the mailbox. I cannot take it out. I called the post office and spoke to the supervisor in charge of carriers. He told me he would talk to the carrier.

The next day, the box was still in the mailbox. I had to call the post office again. The supervisor told me she would leave a note for the carrier to take it out of the box and leave it by my door. Is this ridiculous or what?

I spoke to the carrier. He apologized. He did not want to leave it by the door. He did not think when he dropped it in that I would have trouble removing it.

The post office has done it again! In four months, they lost four to five envelopes. Two contained checks, one was a letter I wanted a tenant to drop in the slot in my former building, and another was a small manila padded envelope containing pictures being returned from an Illinois based company. The response from an employee at the Post Office? She said, "I am sorry." I posed the question, "Do I have to start sending everything certified mail? I should not have to send it certified." She told me, "No."

I asked the company to pay for the pictures which they mailed from their headquarters. Maybe the package did not even get to the post office. How do I know that nobody stole it because they

liked the pictures so much. The company would not pay for it. I
said until it reached the postal carrier, they were responsible. I
told them that I would not buy anything from them. They lost a
good customer for a mere $20.00. Is that stupid or what? The
excuse was they did not solicit the pictures from me. Maybe so,
but they did accept them to look at what I had, probably knowing
they would never buy them.

Well, the post office has done it again. Of course, they blamed
it on the company's packaging. It was an oversized envelope. One
would think, since the post office spent thousands of dollars on
sorting equipment, the equipment would spit something out that
was too big for it. Of course not. It chewed it up and chewed up
the bumper sticker I ordered.

I told the company's employees what happened. The employees sent the sticker in the same envelope and the same amount of
stamps. It arrived in one piece.

I tried to get satisfaction from the post office. Yeah, right! I got
excuses, lectures, and condescending and patronizing statements,
not just from an employee but also from a manager in Consumer
Affairs. I sent letters to Senators Boxer and Feinstein and Congressman Schiff. I said I was tired of long lines, bad interpersonal
skills, condescending and patronizing attitudes, and the excuses. I
also told them if the post office was a regular company, I would
have dumped them for lousy service a long time ago.

You do not have to be a caregiver to be frustrated with the post
office. A lot of people are frustrated and have written letters to the
editor of various newspapers.

On a different matter, Title 3B, a County program, cut hours
from 16 to 8 hours a month. The County is running low on funds.
What a time to cut the hours. While I moved, I needed all the
help I could get. The County is returning 8 hours for the month
of January and then who knows. It seems the County, like many
caregivers, is taking one step at a time. I understand I am getting
the 8 hours for February.

I asked for and received expanded hours on IHSS so I could

get a little more money since taking care of my father has become a more difficult job. This helped. Now, if Medi-Cal was that easy. Only time will tell.

My father received his statement of earnings from Social Security. They sent it to the former address. I called Social Security a month ago to report our change of address.

I hate dealing with the government with a passion. Since my father is eligible for IHSS and pays a share of cost, he can receive Medi-Cal without another share of cost.

I called the Department of Public Social Services office in Sylmar. The employee referred me to another number in Glendale. I called the number the employee gave me. The employee who answered the phone told me since I did not have a worker, I had to call another number which she gave me. I called that number and the employee sent me back to the number I had just called.

I hung up the phone and I dialed the number and asked to speak to a supervisor. I told the supervisor what happened. She told me she would put an application in the mail.

Now, what was so difficult that either employee could not send me an application? I do not know. Talk about lousy customer service! I became angry.

After I hung up, I called my County Supervisor's field office. I told his representative what transpired. She said she would report it to the appropriate people and apologized.

As a family caregiver, speaker, author, chief cook, and bottle washer, I do not have time to run around chasing wild geese.

It turns out I did not need an application since I went through IHSS. However, there is a problem with Medi-Cal. For some reason, the State of California's computers spit it out. Nobody knows why this is happening. Someone gave me several numbers. I called one and it just rang and rang and rang. I called another which was the data center in Sacramento. They referred me to Human Services. The Automated Response Unit referred me to the County. After that, I said "Enough is enough."

I placed a call to the County Supervisor's field office and asked for their help even though there is nothing listed in the County's computers.

My next call was to my Assemblymember's office. An employee told me someone would handle it next week. Nobody handled it. In fact, there was not even a file jacket made up as they are supposed to do for constituents who call into the office.

It is a good thing we are not totally dependent on this card, though it would be nice to have Medi-Cal cover a bath chair and incontinence supplies

Since the in-home agency and I will be parting company at the end of the month, I tried to find out how to keep my Title 3B hours. Eventually, as you will see, I found the answer for at least March and April.

My social worker is very nice and understanding. All social workers, whether or not they work for the government, should be understanding and compassionate. Unfortunately, they are not, as you can see by my information listed below.

I left a message for the person I thought was still the Regional Administrator on my list. She actually is in the San Gabriel Valley area. She did not call back but she gave it to an on-duty worker. Supposedly all she gave the worker was my phone number. The on-duty worker called, and the situation went downhill from there. I sure would like to know from where the government hires its employees. She said she did not know anything about Title 3B. She kept interrupting me and told me I was getting overpaid by getting the 8 hours from Title 3B. It seems she believed I was cheating the system. Let her try living my life. I do not think she would make that assumption anymore.

I told her I wanted to talk to her supervisor. She said, "Okay, you can call" and then hung up on me.

I placed my second call to the Regional Administrator's voice mail. This time, the Deputy Administrator returned the call. I told her what happened. She apologized and said she would talk to the employee and the Regional Administrator about the incident.

I made my third call to my County Supervisor's field office. The employee gave me the number for the downtown office. I called the downtown office and reported the incident. The employee said she would do some research and let me know.

The next day, I received a call from the Deputy Administrator. They had placed it back in the lap of the Department of Public Social Services.

Eventually, the in-home agency got it together. They will pay me for March and April under Title 3B. I will turn around and pay the aides who come to help me.

The Medi-Cal problem should be resolved. However, it was a hairy few days. The State employees referred back to the County. What a mess.

I called the County Supervisor's office and the employee told me, "They are working on it." I gave her the name of the State employee and told her to pass on the message to call him in Sacramento.

My dad's social worker from IHSS called. The problem should be resolved and they had a lot of people working on the case. My dad's social worker from IHSS is great.

Caregivers, the trick is to find a social worker who actually cares about the people he or she services. In order to find a great social worker, you may have to fight a little or go to the top. However, remember you are still dealing with a government that is steeped in red tape and bureaucracy. Government or not, there are some "duds" out there who never should be social workers.

Considering all of the problems that I have had with the Medi-Cal system, I would be screaming my head off just about now. It is now two weeks and I have not received my father's card. I did receive a letter stating that the State of CA would pay my father's Medicare deduction. It is a start, at least.

I placed another call to the County Board of Supervisor's field office and another to my Assemblymember. I hope one of these offices can resolve this nonsense. It is a good thing that my father is not relying on just Medicare or Medi-Cal because we would be up a creek without a paddle.

I did not just have problems with the Medi-Cal system or trying to obtain dad's card. One day, someone from the Department of Public Social Services called me and wanted to talk to my dad. I explained that my dad had dementia and I had Power of Attorney. This employee did not care. The employee said that she could not talk to me because it was a matter of confidentiality. I managed to get, "We are working on the problem" out of the employee. For this, I was hassled.

The former division chief contacted me today regarding my letter to the County Supervisor. That was fast. I sent it on April 11, 2001. Today is April 17, 2001.

He apologized only approximately four times. He is very astute and could hear the frustration in my letter. He said he would take care of the situation and agreed that the employee had carried the confidentiality issue too far. In regard to the Medi-Cal card, he said he would turn it over to the Deputy Administrator. He said it was not a County problem. I told him I called my Assemblymember's office as well because nobody seemed to get anywhere with Sacramento. He said he would call me on Thursday. In the meantime, my social worker called to let me know that the Assembly member's staff called her regarding the problem.

I hope that I do not have to call all over creation to get this resolved. My next stop will be my State Senator and a consumer TV advocate.

Will miracles never cease? My social worker called in the morning to let me know that my father's Medi-Cal looked as if it was up and running and to test it. While I was out running errands, I did just that. According to the phone call one of the pharmacy technicians made to the Medi-Cal eligibility number, my father is eligible and on the system. All I need is his card.

After I returned home, I placed a call to the social worker and gave her the information. After I hung up with her, the Deputy Administrator called to say he was in the system. I told her how I tested it. She promised to work on getting my father his card.

Approximately, forty-five minutes after she called me, the former division chief called. I told him what transpired and he told me it was a very good sign. I quickly added, "Now if I can only get the card." He told me that if I still needed help to call him. I said, "Okay." I will call the appropriate people tomorrow and thank them for their help.

Hooray! I finally received dad's Medi-Cal card on April 23, 2001. Yeah! Now, I can start looking into new doctors for him.

Caregivers, sometimes you have to go over peoples' heads and become very assertive to obtain desired results.

On another matter concerning the government, I contacted Fair Housing/HUD regarding the incident with our former landlord. Customer service was so lousy, I wrote my Federal representatives and asked that someone do customer service training.

The employee from HUD called and said, "I'm working on your case." I said, "I do not have time to talk to you right now. I am running out the door." She sarcastically replied, "I'm calling about your case, if you do not have time to talk." I interrupted her right then and there.

I told her that it was not that I did not have the time to talk, but it was because I could not take the time to talk. I explained that I am a family caregiver and that I had to do errands while I had someone watching my dad. She insisted. I told her not to "cop an attitude" with me. She told me, "If anybody is copping an attitude, it is you." I asked for her supervisor.

He could use a little customer service training himself. He told me he was sorry but then negated that apology by making an excuse for the employee's anxiety. He told me that higher ups were exerting pressure on employees to close cases in 20 days.

This is not my problem. It is the government's problem. I

explained that he needs to contact the "powers that be" and let them know attitude comes from the top and trickles down level by level by level. I also told him they need to read my first, book, "Do Managers Really Know How To Manage?" I added this information to the letters I sent to my Congressman and my Senators.

I called the Social Security Administration regarding my father's Social Security payments. I become so tired about monitoring phone calls to provide quality service. Employees in the government delivering quality service? That is the biggest joke I ever heard with some exceptions, of course.

Anyway, I was connected to an employee who became argumentative. She needed to talk to my father. I told her that he has dementia. She insisted talking to him. I asked her what part of "he has dementia" did she not understand. I told her I have power of attorney. She insisted. I told her I wanted to speak to a supervisor. She asked, "Why do you need a supervisor? They are not going to change anything." I asked for her name. She said, "I gave it to you at the beginning of the conversation." I said "Give it to me again." She did not even have a clue.

I hung up on her, took a very long time to get connected and finally spoke to a supervisor. I told her my experience and added if one is giving bad service, others are doing it as well. She agreed. However, she still quoted me the Privacy Act and told me (even though I gave her the amounts) she could not confirm the amounts and to go back to the bank. This is utterly ridiculous.

I learned that the employee at the bank screwed up and gave me incorrect information. I called a supervisor at the bank and informed her of the situation. I also told her I questioned the amount of the ACH deposit. She never took it one step further. The supervisor apologized. I did not want anything. I just wanted her to be informed because of the lack of customer service, follow through and attention to detail.

Yes, dealing with the government is one source still causing a lot of frustration and stress. Most family caregivers have limited

budgets and have to deal with government agencies. I wish somebody would make things simpler for us. Legislators, are you listening? I can only hope.

Now onto Chapter Nine—Comments Better Left Unsaid

CHAPTER NINE

COMMENTS BETTER LEFT UNSAID

I do not mind people's comments when they say, "Bless You" or "God Bless You." I usually answer, "Thank you. I need all the help I can get."

People also say, "You are a good daughter." I reply, "I try." However, there are times when I do not feel I am "a good daughter."

I find it difficult to believe that I am a good daughter when I lose my patience with my father. I am not the only caregiver to feel this way.

Other comments better left unsaid are, "Why don't you put your father in a home?" or "How can you work or have a life if you do not put your father in a home?"

The woman who posed the "Why" question is not a caregiver. She made a statement based on her experience of helping a friend who was about to be placed in a home.

I just looked at her. Talking about the placement of a friend is not the same as placing a parent who raised, diapered, helped me and soothed my mountain of tears when I fell down, got hurt, etc.

People who ask the "Why" question do not have a clue as to the bond I still have with my father, although I do not have an idea as to how long I will last as his family caregiver.

The person who made the other comment was a caregiver. She placed her mother in a nursing home. Several months later, the mother died. Once she placed her mother in a home, the mother gave up and refused to eat.

I believe my father would lose his fighting spirit. He said if he did not have me, he would give up and die. I believe him.

I replied, "If I placed him, he would give up and die." She just shrugged her shoulders.

I would think that a family caregiver would be more compassionate and supportive.

Obviously, I am not ready to sign my father's death warrant. His death will come soon enough.

I realize that some people might say some of the comments out of concern. However, that is not the way to show it. Another person I met gave me money even though I did not ask. She periodically made comments that were better left unsaid. She told me, "Just put your father in a home and get a life." One day, I mentioned this to her and I told her I did not like what she said. She said okay and that she would watch what she said in the future. She said the reason she made that remark was because I was feeling very stressed out and she thought it would be helpful. How could anybody think that telling me to put my father in a home and get a life would not be stressful? She made one more remark I did not like. She gave me money for which I did not ask. Then she said she could not "pay" for both me and her. Who asked her? Shortly, after this incident, I wrote her a note and said I did not want to see her anymore. This woman was supposed to be a friend of mine. Not in my book!

In my first chapter I also voiced concerns due to the comments made by the paramedics that came to take care of my dad.

I would like medical professionals and those at the HMO to stop trying to convince me to place my father. They should be trying to help me, not hinder me. But then, if I placed him, they would not have to deal with him anymore. People like my father cost HMO's money because Medicare does not pay them enough.

While my dad and I were waiting for the wheelchair to arrive so I could wheel him out, I met a woman who began to talk. She asked me what was wrong with my father so I told her.

The woman's next comment was one of those that are "better

left unsaid." I cannot remember everything she said but she did say with certainty, "He is not going to live too much longer." I expect this may be true, but one never knows.

Nevertheless, that is a hell of a comment to make! Sometimes people are such morons, I cannot stand it.

I have a friend who means well but she needs to also stop making comments better left unsaid. We talked today about work, caregiving, money, etc. She said to me, "You do not have to answer this if you do not want to, but what are you going to do when your father dies?" I said, "I hope everything I am working on sells." She told me she would pray for me. She has asked this question too many times. Once was bad enough, but not three or four times.

I guess when my father dies and if my ship has not come in yet, I will be out on the street.

She still has not come over because she is too busy working. However, after she had an operation, I took her grocery shopping, and drove her home the time she came over to visit me at my former apartment.

I just wish people would help by assisting me with whatever I need them to do, buy my items, validate and show compassion instead of saying comments better left unsaid.

Now onto Chapter Ten—Employers: Do They Really Know How To Manage?

CHAPTER TEN

EMPLOYERS: DO THEY REALLY KNOW HOW TO MANAGE?

In my original book, "A Daughter's Lament: The Trials and Tribulations of a Family Caregiver," I mentioned the importance of giving family caregivers a little leeway in regard to their jobs.

In my management book, "Do Managers Really Know How To Manage?/How to Lose or Keep a Good Hardworking Employee," I wrote about the importance of positive employer/employee relations, giving praise, giving the employee the tools to do the job, etc.

Employers need to assist employees, especially those who are caregivers.

How do you think any employee feels when you constantly criticize the employee, especially one who is a family caregiver. Do you want to destroy morale, productivity, etc.? Any employee will have lower morale, productivity, self-esteem, etc., if you continue on your present path.

I returned to work part-time as a marketing director for a nursing home. I started in January 2001 and I only came into the office one to two days a week. Obtaining results is difficult enough without the boss constantly telling me just how low our census is. Three months later, the job was over. It was on a trial basis. Of course, the administrator made some comments as if I was too busy to achieve results due to caregiving duties. No, that was not it. It was a combination of a lot of other things that were out of my control.

There was a lack of patients and the discharge planners and families wanted a facility close by so they could visit without problems. These are only a few of the problems that were driving the census down.

Do not add to employee stress by constantly reminding the employee that the employee is not doing enough to obtain results. You are going to alienate your employee in the process.

I do not understand the logic in the situation listed below but it does not paint a very favorable view of the company.

The facility in which I worked as marketing director terminated me effective April 8, 2001. This is on a Sunday, I might add, and not even the cut-off date for payroll. However, I made a commitment to bringing lunch to one of the hospitals. I persuaded the administrator to make April 11, 2001, my last day.

I received my other check from the previous pay period which stated it was the final check. It definitely was not the final check and I let them know that right off the bat. The date of the check was April 3, 2001. The end of the pay period was March 31, 2001. Go figure!

First, the secretary who also does payroll told me I was actually paid up to April 1, 2001, not March 31, 2001.

Second, they did not know how many hours I would end up working my last day. This was the reason for not having my final check on hand.

Third, the secretary told me the check was marked a final check because 4/01/01 was included in the date and before I spoke to the administrator.

My original termination date was April 8th. So, how could they mark it a final check when I worked the first week of April, the pay period was five days prior to the original termination date, and people knew my termination date?

They informed me on April 3, 2001 that my termination date was April 8, 2001. Will someone please explain the logic in this mess? I do not see it.

Also, the administrator told me they let me go because I could not produce patients, as if it was my fault for the census falling. However, another department head told me that they terminated me because they needed someone there everyday.

Sure, they needed someone to be a receptionist, answer the phones, and perform general office duties. They need a general office person to do this work, not the marketing director, and certainly not if they wanted the marketing director to produce.

The day after I started, I asked the administrator if I could bring my father into the facility during the hours I was supposed to work. After all, it is a nursing home. They could watch him during the hours I was out in the field and then I could take him home when I left.

The administrator told me that the corporate office wanted to see results before they gave out perks. The company has it backwards. Since I was part time and did not receive benefits, this was one "benefit" the corporation should have allowed. If they did, I could have come in and been the employee they obviously wanted. Of course, maybe I would have hated it since I hate being tied down to a desk.

At my interview, I told the administrator about my first book on employer/employee relations. He said that maybe I could teach them a thing or two. I did not think so at that time, but after constantly hearing how low was the census and not being able to get that one perk, I do now. I had planned on contacting the main office. The only problem is that so far I cannot find the address for the corporate office. I find that very interesting.

Maybe some employers need to learn how to really manage.

Now onto Chapter Eleven—The Closing Chapter

CHAPTER ELEVEN

THE CLOSING CHAPTER

When I started this sequel, I did not know how long it would take me to write it. However, there is so much happening, this sequel just continued to grow.

Therefore, I have decided to start writing the third volume. I do not know how fast I can write it, what is going to happen to my father, etc. I would like to do the third segment as there is a lot more to tell. I hope I am given the chance to continue.

I have more than 30,000 words of the new book written. The third and final installment will have something the original and the sequel do not. It will have helpful websites where caregivers can go to find help.

After reading this sequel and the original book, I hope you have come away with a greater understanding of what it means to be a family caregiver to someone who is cognitively impaired.

Watch for Volume 3 coming in 2003.

####